LIFE MANAGEMENT SKILLS VII

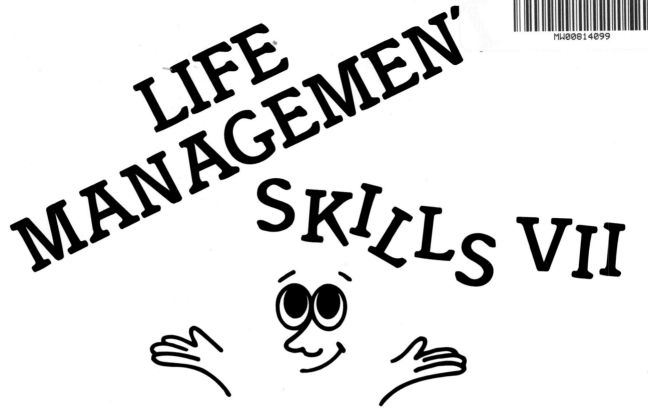

reproducible activity handouts created for facilitators

A sampler collection of...

Activities of Daily Living	Leisure	Responsibility
Anxiety	Money Management	Self-Esteem
Communication	Productive / Work Activities	Skill Development
Coping Skills	Recovery	Social Skills
Emotions	Relapse Prevention	Spirituality
Goals	Relationships	Time Management

Kathy L. Korb-Khalsa, OTR/L   Estelle A. Leutenberg

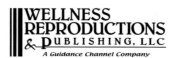
WELLNESS REPRODUCTIONS & PUBLISHING, LLC
A Guidance Channel Company

© 2002 Wellness Reproductions and Publishing, LLC • 800 / 669-9208 • FAX 800 / 501-8120 • www.wellness-resources.com

We celebrate being open to life's possibilities . . .
including treasured family relationships.

We dedicate this book to

THE GALLEN FAMILY

Mel, Sue Young, John and Ryan
Harvey and Harriet
Robert, Jennifer Willford and Elisabeth
Ellen, David and Jessi Krupnick

Special thanks to the following therapists, counselors and educators,
whose submissions of activity handouts for Life Management Skills VII were selected.
The Facilitator's Information Sheet on the back of each handout
has a box with information identifying the submitter.

*The Roman numerals listed after some of the submitter's names indicate other books
in the Life Management Skills series for which handouts were also contributed.*

Courtney Behrens Bolduc, OTR/L

Nicole Bilodeau Shea, MOT, OTR/L

Enid Chung, B.A.

Tamara Cole, CTRS

Erica Pond Clements, O.T. Reg (Ont.),
  Dip. Add. [IV, V, VI]

Nancy Day, BScO.T. Reg (Ont.) [V, VI]

Sherrie L. Easton, LMSW

Diana Fain, MOT, OTR/L

Dominique G. Fifi, M.S., CADC III, CCSII, CPC, CGC

April Folsom, APPCM

Rick Germann, MA, LCPC, RPRP [VI]

Marty Golub, CTRS [V, VI, VI]

Cherie A. Johnson, MOTR/L

K. Oscar Larson, OTL, MA, BCG [IV, V, VI]

Beth Lucas, OTR/L

Mark S. Macko, M.Ed. [V]

Elana Blachman Markovitz, M.A., OTR/L [VI]

Esterlee Molyneux, MS, SSW [V]

Sandra Netto-Marceau, MSW, LICSW [V, VI]

Kathleen O' Neill, COTA/L

Roberta J. Ott, COTA, M.Ed. [V, VI]

Jodi Wilson Overstreet, M.Ed., LPC, NCC

Kathy L. Parker, COTA/L

Joan Rascati, A.S. Human Services [V, VI]

Katie Schroeder-Smith, MOT

Nina Beth Sellner, M.Ed. [V]

Donald Shields, BRE, MTS, CAPPE [VI]

Mary K. Tilden-Walker, BSW, LSW [V]

Robert L. Vitelli, MS, Public Administration

Betty A. Welch, Ph.D. [V, VI]

Kimberly White, CTRS

Paul D. Zavala, MOT

FOREWORD

The inspiration for our LIFE MANAGEMENT SKILLS books originated from an ongoing practical need observed within a mental health setting. Handouts had been typically used in treatment as a launching pad for activities, an organizational tool, a visual aid, a tangible reminder of information presented, and as a method for building rapport. However, available handouts often did not meet necessary, high-quality standards in content desired, format, appearance and organization – and lacked permission for reproduction.

We have attempted to meet these standards by offering this sampler collection of handouts which are highly reproducible, organized in a logical manner, designed for specific well-defined purposes, and activity-based, allowing for extensive client involvement. The graphic representations are intentionally different from handout to handout in typestyle, art and design to increase visual appeal, provide variety and clarify meaning.

LIFE MANAGEMENT SKILLS handouts are adaptable and have a broad usage enabling therapists, social workers, nurses, teachers, psychologists, counselors and other professionals to focus on specific goals with their specified populations.

The book has been designed to offer reproducible handouts on the front of each page and nonreproducible facilitator's information on the reverse side. The Facilitator's Information Sheet includes the following sections: Purpose, General Comments and Possible Activities.

We specifically chose spiral binding to allow for easier and accurate reproduction, an especially white paper for clear, sharp copies, and a heavier paper stock for its durability and opacity. If adaptations to any of the handouts are desired, it is recommended to make one copy of the handout, include the changes which will meet *your* specific needs, and then use this copy as the original.

We hope that you will find these handouts in LIFE MANAGEMENT SKILLS VII fun, innovative and informative. We wish you much success with your therapeutic and educational endeavors and hope we can continue to be of assistance. Remember... creative handouts will hopefully generate creative activities and contribute to a greater sense of WELLNESS!

Wellness Reproductions and Publishing, LLC

Kathy L. Korb-Khalsa

Estelle A. Leutenberg

THANK YOU TO AMY LEUTENBERG BRODSKY, LISW

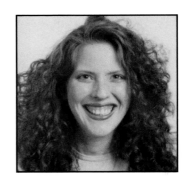

our Wellness Reproductions and Publishing artist, whose creativity and skill as an illustrator, and experience with clients, continues to give the Life Management Skills books unique, humorous and meaningful artwork, and whose insights from her clinical work offered guidance on the content as well. Amy received her Masters of Science in Social Administration from the Mandel School of Applied Social Sciences, Case Western Reserve University. Her art training was received at Kent State University where she achieved a BFA in Studio Art. She continues to pursue her career as an artist, as well as facilitating wellness with children and families in crisis.

WELLNESS REPRODUCTIONS AND PUBLISHING, LLC

is an innovative company which began in 1988. As developers of creative therapeutic and educational products, we have a strong commitment to the mental health profession. Our rapidly growing business began by authoring and self-publishing the book LIFE MANAGEMENT SKILLS I. We have extended our product line to include group presentation posters, therapeutic games, skill building cards, EMOTIONS© identification products, LIFE MANAGEMENT SKILLS II, III, IV, V, VI, VII, SEALS (Self-Esteem and Life Skills) books and corresponding cards, Self-Reflections and Images of Wellness Print series and educational products about serious mental illness. Our books are created with feedback from our customers. Please refer to the last page of this book, our 'FEEDBACK' page, and let us hear from YOU!

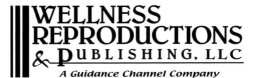

A Guidance Channel Company

P.O. Box 760 • Plainview, New York 11803-0760
800 / 669-9208 • FAX 800 / 501-8120
email: info@wellness-resources.com • www.wellness-resources.com

TABLE OF CONTENTS - by Topic

Page numbers are on the Facilitator's Information Sheet, located on the reverse side of each handout.

Presentation Poster, Handout Pads and Note Pads available (see order form - last page) [over for Table of Contents - by Activity Handout]

TABLE OF CONTENTS - by Activity Handout

Page numbers are on the Facilitator's Information Sheet, located on the reverse side of each handout.

Presentation Poster, Handout Pads and Note Pads available (see order form - last page) [over for Table of Contents - by Activity Handout]

GETTING THINGS DONE

during times of illness

One daily task or activity I am able to do is…

_____

_____

_____

What enables or helps me to do this is…

_____

_____

_____

One daily task or activity I feel unable to do is…

_____

_____

_____

Strategies that could help me to do this task are …

_____

_____

_____

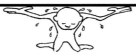

GETTING THINGS DONE
during times of illness

I. PURPOSE:

To discover strategies for accomplishing daily tasks.

II. GENERAL COMMENTS:

For individuals with mental illness, even small daily tasks can be very difficult. This can feel quite distressing and overwhelming. This exercise focuses initially on a task they are able to accomplish so that factors which enable them can be identified. By identifying strategies such as breaking tasks into smaller, more manageable steps, participants can then explore how to apply these to tasks which are more overwhelming and difficult to tackle.

III. POSSIBLE ACTIVITIES:

A. 1. Ask participants to share one task they were able to accomplish today prior to coming to group no matter how small. Facilitate a brief discussion on the importance of achieving and acknowledging small accomplishments throughout the day.

2. Distribute handouts and pens.

3. Instruct participants to complete the first box. Allow for some sharing from participants regarding the strategies that enable them to accomplish small tasks, e.g., task is simple, task is a part of daily routine, encouragement or help from another.

4. Instruct participants to complete the second box. Allow sufficient time to discuss possible strategies that would assist them in tackling some of the more difficult tasks.
Look for ideas such as:
   - breaking tasks into small manageable steps
   - working on one step at a time
   - setting a goal of only 10 minutes or so at first
   - giving positive and supportive self-talk
   - taking breaks and pacing self
   - rewarding self for small efforts
   - avoiding a perfectionistic approach

5. Conclude by having participants identify and share a goal to accomplish a task (or part of a task) which they have found difficult to try.

B. 1. Distribute handouts and pens and divide group into pairs.

2. Instruct pairs to interview each other with the questions on the handout. Writing can be optional. Allow sufficient time.

3. Reconvene. Have pairs report to the large group strategies for getting things done which they learned from each other in B.2. List on flipchart.

4. Facilitate discussion on ways group members might motivate or encourage each other to accomplish some of the daily tasks participants are finding too difficult to get done. This works especially well if participants are taking part in a continuing group program.

5. Keep flipchart posted throughout day / week and refer to it as a visual reminder of helpful suggestions.

Activity handout and facilitator's information submitted by Nancy Day, BScO.T. Reg (Ont), Markham, Ontario, Canada. Nancy has had 20 of her handouts published in the Life Management Skills series. She provides hospital-based occupational therapy services to clients experiencing mental health problems within a team-oriented program emphasizing group therapies. Nancy's leisure interests are quilting, reading, antiques and hiking.

How I Can Improve My Body Image and be My PERSONAL BEST

"I will be the best I can be from head to toe."

In our society, there is pressure to present an image of near physical perfection. Since this is impossible to achieve, we often suffer from low self-esteem and/or have a negative body image.

Part of maturing is to accept our limitations and to take responsibility for making the most of what we have. Take a look at yourself from head to toe and determine if you are doing what you can to be YOUR PERSONAL BEST.

			YES	NO	NOT APPLICABLE
Hair	1.	Washed	☐	☐	☐
	2.	Good haircut	☐	☐	☐
	3.	Neatly combed	☐	☐	☐
Teeth	1.	Brushed	☐	☐	☐
	2.	Flossed	☐	☐	☐
	3.	Fresh breath	☐	☐	☐
Face	1.	Clean	☐	☐	☐
	2.	Makeup	☐	☐	☐
	3.	Aftershave	☐	☐	☐
	4.	Smile	☐	☐	☐
Body	1.	Clean	☐	☐	☐
	2.	Flattering clothes	☐	☐	☐
	3.	Exercise	☐	☐	☐
	4.	Good nutrition	☐	☐	☐
Nails	1.	Clean	☐	☐	☐
	2.	Cut	☐	☐	☐
	3.	Filed smooth	☐	☐	☐

How I Can Improve My Body Image
and be
My PERSONAL BEST

I. PURPOSE:

To identify areas of self-care that have strengths and deficits.

To improve personal appearances and self-image.

II. GENERAL COMMENTS:

It is useful to evaluate if we are taking care of our bodies, and to develop habits which help us to truly appear as the best we can be – therefore improving our self-image.

III. POSSIBLE ACTIVITIES:

A. 1. Circulate relevant magazines (fashion, sports, women's, men's), calendars and posters among group members.

   2. Ask group members to look at these publications and to discuss how society pressures us through the printed word as well as in photographs, television, movies, etc., to look like a perfect "10".

   3. Distribute handouts and pencils.

   4. Give group members several minutes to place a check mark under YES, NO or NOT APPLICABLE, evaluating how they are caring for themselves. Ask them to consider how they look and present themselves to others.

   5. Have group members share their findings.

   6. Discuss ways in which they can improve our outward appearance.

B. 1. Distribute handouts and pencils.

   2. Ask group members to complete by checking YES, NO or NOT APPLICABLE after each category.

   3. Look at the YES checks and the NO checks to determine areas in which group members can improve their appearance.

   4. Discuss techniques and products group members use to help keep themselves looking their best.

   5. Discuss how our appearance affects our day-to-day life and how improving our looks enhances our self-image.

   6. If available, give 'goodies' at the end of the group: free samples of shampoo, toothpaste, perfume, fancy soap, nail file, etc. as a boost to begin work in these areas. (Staff can collect from hotels when on vacation.)

Activity handout and facilitator's information submitted by Roberta J. Ott, COTA, M.Ed., Allentown, PA.
Roberta is a Therapeutic Activity Services Worker, providing programs to adult psychiatric patients, e.g., arts, crafts, music, coping skills and life skill development as well as community trips to prepare for discharge. Her leisure interests are tole painting and reading.

Oral Hygiene

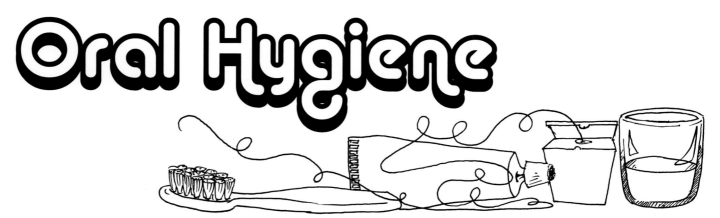

Name _____

Write a brief description of how you care for your teeth and gums:

_____

_____

_____

Are these statements True or False?   (T or F)

____ Brushing your teeth everyday causes cavities and tooth decay.

____ Brushing your teeth helps prevent bad breath.

____ Brushing your teeth will not prevent gum disease.

____ Brushing your teeth can help make food taste better.

____ Flossing teeth removes extra food that is caught between teeth and helps prevent gum disease.

____ Dentures should be kept clean just as much as teeth.

Put a check (✓) if you...

____ Use a good quality, soft bristled toothbrush

____ Brush teeth in a circular motion

____ Brush teeth at least 2 times a day

____ Use toothpaste you like

____ Use dental floss

____ Brush each tooth inside and out

____ See your dental hygienist every 6 months

____ Rinse your mouth with water or mouthwash

____ Brush surface of tongue to fight bad breath

____ Use abrasives, powders or acid cleansers to clean dentures

____ Other _____

Oral Hygiene

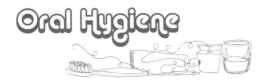

I. PURPOSE:
To increase awareness of techniques and benefits of proper oral hygiene.

II. GENERAL COMMENTS:
A wide variety of factors such as depression, wanting to distance oneself from others, lack of education, side effects of medications and psychosis, may contribute to the lack of oral hygiene often observed by health care professionals. An action-oriented approach that will introduce this topic honestly and with dignity may promote the awareness needed to improve this important life skill for the client as well as those around him/her.

III. POSSIBLE ACTIVITIES:
A. 1. Introduce topic and distribute handouts and pens/pencils.
   2. Ask group members to write a brief description about oral hygiene.
   3. Answer six True/False questions: (1)T, (2)T, (3)F, (4)T, (5)T, (6)T and discuss as needed.
   4. As a group, complete the checklist and share answers by explaining the steps used for good oral hygiene.
   5. Ask group members what the benefits are for good oral hygiene.
   6. Offer reinforcements, such as trial toothpaste or toothbrushes to participants.

B. 1. Introduce topic and as a warm-up, ask group members to identify the toothpaste they prefer.
   2. Ask group members what obstacles they are facing in taking good oral care. Offer a few ideas if the group seems resistant and write on board:
       a. No money to go to dentist
       b. Afraid it will hurt
       c. Too depressed to even take care of the details
   3. Create atmosphere of understanding and recognize all responses as valid. Explain that towards the end of the session, the group might offer suggestions on how to overcome these obstacles.
   4. Next, ask group members to list benefits of proper oral hygiene and list on board.
   5. Distribute handouts and give group members ten minutes to complete.
   6. Discuss all sections thoroughly. See A.3. above for answers to True/False questions.
   7. Revisit list of obstacles to good oral hygiene and problem-solve, as a group, any possible suggestions to remove obstacles.
   8. Discuss possibility of goal setting or checklists serving as methods to improve this life skill.
   9. Offer reinforcements to participants, such as trial toothpaste or toothbrushes.

Activity handout and facilitator's information submitted by Cherie A. Johnson, MOTR/L, Miami, FL.
Cherie works with both children and adults with various diagnosis from autism, developmental delays, cerebral palsy, Davis syndrome to orthopedic injuries.
For leisure, she enjoys scrapbooking, growing orchids, needlepoint crafts, bike riding and swimming.

Anxiety Disorder Biography

by _____

Prepare a biography of your Anxiety Disorder.
Write a chronological history of your disorder, the feelings you have had,
and the effect your disorder has had on your life and members of your family.

1. When did the disorder first begin? _____

2. Was the onset gradual or sudden? _____

3. Has the disorder been constantly present or do the symptoms come and go? _____

4. Have you had times when you were completely free of it since the first time it appeared? _____
   Please give details of this if you can. _____
   _____

5. When did you know the name or diagnosis of the disorder that you have? _____

6. How severe has your disorder been at its very worst? (Circle)

   Terrible 0   1   2   3   4   5   6   7   8   9   10 Not problematic at all

7. What has been the major negative effect(s) on your life? _____

8. What particular things do you avoid? _____

9. Have you ever felt particularly low, blue, or depressed?   Yes _____   No _____

10. If you have felt depressed, is it because of your fears – that is, do your fears and the effects
    of your fears cause you to feel depressed or does your depression come on even when you are
    not fearful? _____

11. Do you know of anyone in your family that has had similar problems? Who? _____

12. Have you been on any medications for anxiety?   Yes _____   No _____

13. If yes, when did you receive them, from whom and what effects did they have? _____
    _____

14. How much alcohol do you use? _____   How often? _____

15. Do you ever drink in order to treat your fears? _____

16. How much do you smoke? _____

Please add any other things that you wish to this biography.

_____
_____
_____

Anxiety Disorder Biography

I. **PURPOSE:**
To provide the history and details of the anxiety disorder for the client and the health care professional(s).

II. **GENERAL COMMENTS:**
An accurate history of any disorder is helpful in fully understanding the client. At times, it is wise to take a step back and get perspective of the duration and patterns associated with the disorder. This activity can be helpful for staff to assess motivation and provide valuable information to report to the team. This activity will help clients normalize their experiences by collecting their thoughts, having a 'place to put them' and sharing them if appropriate.

III. **POSSIBLE ACTIVITIES:**
A. 1. Discuss importance of knowing about one's disorder and diagnosis.
2. Distribute handouts and pens.
3. Give group 15 minutes to complete.
4. Collect all handouts to review later.
5. Ask group members if they gained any insights from completing the handouts and to share if appropriate.
6. Invite a guest to speak about successful anxiety management.
7. Process event with group members, focussing on helpful strategies to manage this disorder.
8. After group, review handouts, collect needed information and return to group members.

B. 1. Explain to group members that due to the discomfort of discussing mental illnesses, many people feel that they are the only ones with certain symptoms. As society removes the stigmas around mental illnesses, it is hopeful to think that people will be able to discuss symptoms, illnesses and treatment in a safe environment.
2. Discuss what a safe environment is and is not. With whom is it safe to talk about these things? Under what circumstances? What are the benefits?
3. Explain that today's group is for sharing. If questions are too uncomfortable, no one needs to share all responses, but it is encouraged to share at least a few thoughts within one's comfort level.
4. Distribute handouts and pens.
5. Give group members 15 minutes to complete.
6. Allow group members to divide into dyads or triads and share as able.
7. Give subgroups ten minutes to disclose anything they choose from the handouts.
8. Reconvene.
9. Provide resources of books, tapes, videos, web sites, a FACT SHEET about anxiety disorders or any other material that will support group members in managing anxiety.
10. Process by asking group members about benefits or gains made through today's participation.

Activity handout and facilitator's information submitted by Dominique G. Fifi, M.S., CADC III, CCSII, CPC, CGC. Dominique has 20 years experience as a mental health and substance abuse therapist specializing in substance abuse, gambling, anxiety disorders, BPD and dual disabilities. She was the first certified gambling counselor in the state of Wisconsin (and possibly the only native Belgian counselor there)! She is now in administration, carrying a small case-load, too. Dominique loves to ride a motorcycle, play piano, read, fish, and play video games!

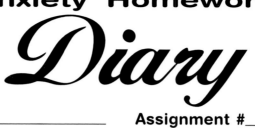

Anxiety Homework
Diary

Name _____   **Assignment #**_____

For period _____ **to** _____

Target behavior _____

Avoidance behavior I usually engage in _____
_____
_____

Target task (exposure) _____

Response prevention (what I did not do when exposed) _____
_____
_____

Before proceeding with behavioral assignment, did I inform my spouse or
significant other of my assignment?   yes _____   no _____

What happened after my exposure?_____
_____
_____

What happened during and/or after when I did not avoid the phobic object
or situation?_____
_____
_____

How do I feel about my assignment?_____

How do I feel about my progress or lack of progress? _____
_____
_____

DISCOMFORT RATINGS

0 ⟵——————————————⟶ 8

NOT BOTHERED   **SEVERELY BOTHERED**

(0-8) before assignment _____   (0-8) during assignment _____   (0-8) after assignment _____

Other comments: _____
_____
_____

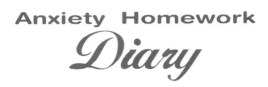

Anxiety Homework Diary

I. PURPOSE:

To facilitate diary-keeping as a way to measure gradual exposure to anxiety-provoking situations.

To reduce avoidance behavior and anxiety level typically associated with target behaviors.

II. GENERAL COMMENTS:

Too often, persons afflicted with anxiety believe that avoidance of anxiety-provoking situations will eliminate their anxiety. In fact, ongoing avoidance of the anxiety-induced avoidance behavior strengthens the avoidance behavior and contributes to an increase in anxiety over time. Secondly, persons suffering from anxiety often feel as if they have become a victim of their anxiety. Individuals believe that they have no 'say' relative to when they experience anxiety. Even the term 'panic attack' suggests that which 'comes out of the blue', with no warning and unpredictably. Individuals consequently feel overwhelmed by the anxiety, and powerless to do anything. This diary can be empowering as it can teach how to control anxiety rather than being controlled by it.

III. POSSIBLE ACTIVITIES:

A. 1. Ask individuals in the group to identify and discuss an event in which they experienced significant anxiety. Have them recall their thoughts and behaviors that occurred before, during and after the event.

2. Discuss how group members might approach the anxiety-provoking situation differently than what has been typical for them in the past.

3. Ask group members to identify a target behavior on which they would like to focus.

4. Distribute handouts.

5. Go through a hypothetical example in which group members will easily be able to relate.

6. Assign group members to complete the handout for the next session.

B. 1. After group members have completed the diary, have each member present his / her diary to the group.

2. Allow time for sharing and support.

3. Discuss means of approaching anxiety-eliciting situations.

4. Encourage continued use of additional handouts for continued growth with or without the use of a counselor / therapist.

Activity handout and facilitator's information submitted by Dominique G. Fifi, M.S., CADC III, CCSII, CPC, CGC.
Dominique has 20 years experience as a mental health and substance abuse therapist specializing in substance abuse, gambling, anxiety disorders, BPD and dual disabilities. She was the first certified gambling counselor in the state of Wisconsin (and possibly the only native Belgian counselor there)! She is now in administration, carrying a small case-load, too. Dominique loves to ride a motorcycle, play piano, read, fish, and play video games!

CHALLENGING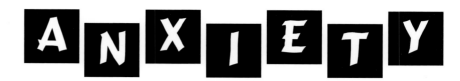

MY ANXIOUS OR FEARFUL THOUGHT:

CHALLENGE IT:

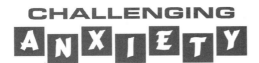
CHALLENGING ANXIETY

I. PURPOSE:

To learn and/or reinforce the skill of challenging or countering anxiety-provoking distortions of thought.

II. GENERAL COMMENTS:

Anxiety is a major symptom experienced by individuals with mental health difficulties. The subjective feeling of anxiety is often fueled by distorted, irrational and/or discouraging thoughts. Many people benefit from finding ways to challenge this nonproductive self-talk. Feedback from peers can be extremely useful in facilitating healthier patterns of thinking.

III. POSSIBLE ACTIVITIES:

A. 1. Have participants share an anxious thought they have had so far today, encouraging them to be as specific as possible.

2. Provide education on the concept that anxious thoughts need to be challenged to promote increased peace of mind. It may be helpful to give some previously prepared examples. One example might be the thought "I probably said the wrong thing to my friend, and that's why she hasn't called me lately." This thought needs to be challenged with "She's likely just really busy – no point in jumping to conclusions which aren't based on reality…we're good friends. If I said something wrong, I'm sure she'd tell me."

3. Distribute handouts and pens. Instruct participants to write their identified anxious thought in the box at the top of the page.

4. Have participants then pass handouts to the person on the right. Each person will then write down a suggestion for challenging the anxious thought, or in other words, a new healthier thought to replace the old one. Continue passing to the right, allowing each fellow participant a few minutes to write another suggestion, until the handout reaches the original writer.

5. Allow time for participants to read their completed handout.

6. Ask for feedback on the effectiveness of the exercise and application of the concept to every day living.

B. 1. Write a list on the flipchart of anxious thoughts, with input from the group, with which they are currently struggling. Ask them to identify any common themes on the list and ask if they relate to the anxious thoughts other participants have identified.

2. Distribute handouts and pens.

3. Instruct group members to write in the top box an anxious thought with which they are struggling and would appreciate help from the group.

4. Divide into sub-groups of three or four. Instruct participants to pass their sheets to each other to receive written feedback on how to challenge and change the identified anxious thought with one that is more calming, rational and/or encouraging.

5. Once participants had a chance to review all the feedback from the other members of their sub-group, reconvene to the large group.

6. Discuss importance of accepting and not dismissing feedback from others.

7. Conclude with discussion on how to use ideas from the session to manage anxiety in every day life.

Activity handout and facilitator's information submitted by Nancy Day, BScO.T. Reg (Ont), Markham, Ontario, Canada. Nancy has had 20 of her handouts published in the Life Management Skills series. She provides hospital-based occupational therapy services to clients experiencing mental health problems within a team-oriented program emphasizing group therapies. Nancy's leisure interests are quilting, reading, antiques and hiking.

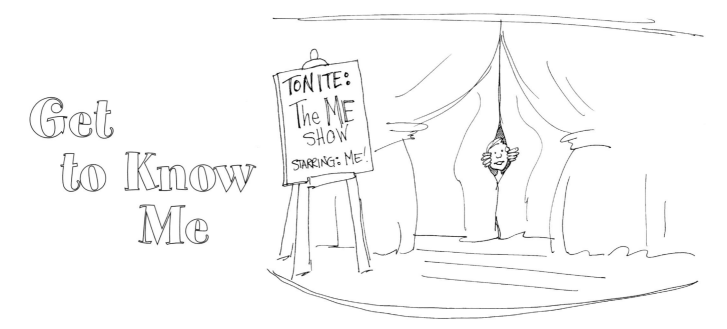

Get to Know Me

If I could go on a trip tomorrow, I would go to _____.

If I could be any animal in the world, I would be _____.

I am proud of myself when _____.

My happiest moment was when _____.

The thing I look forward to the most is _____.

If I could change one thing in my life it would be _____.

If I could change one thing about myself it would be _____.

The thing that makes me the angriest is _____.

My biggest fear is _____.

My saddest moment was when _____.

I feel really bad about myself when _____.

The hardest thing I deal with at home is _____.

The hardest thing I deal with my job or at school is _____.

The most important thing I want you to know about me is _____.

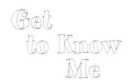
Get
to Know
Me

I. **PURPOSE:**

To develop communication skills and rapport with the people around us.

II. **GENERAL COMMENTS:**

Some of us were taught as children, either verbally or nonverbally, not to talk about ourselves or our feelings. However, the life skill of communicating our emotions enables us to realize important things about ourselves and to feel connected to others.

III. **POSSIBLE ACTIVITIES:**

A. 1. Introduce topic of being able to ask and answer questions as a way of getting to know others and ourselves. Explain that when someone genuinely asks us an interesting question, we need to reflect and answer it honestly. This process of looking inward can be viewed as self-exploration and our response is a disclosure.

   2. Review, if necessary, healthy boundaries for disclosures.

   3. Distribute pens / pencils and handouts.

   4. Give group ten minutes to answer all questions.

   5. Facilitate sharing by asking…
      a. What was the easiest question?
      b. What was the most difficult question?
      c. From what question did you learn the most?
      d. Were the questions in any kind of order? Why do you think that might be?

   6. Divide group into pairs and ask each person to share three of the more interesting disclosures to their partners.

   7. Reconvene and ask group members to process what that was like.

B. 1. Introduce topic of being able to ask and answer questions as a way of getting to know others and ourselves. Explain that when someone genuinely asks us an interesting question, we need to reflect and answer it honestly. This process of looking inward can be viewed as self-exploration and our response is a disclosure.

   2. Review, if necessary, healthy boundaries for disclosures.

   3. Distribute handouts and pens.

   4. Give group fifteen minutes to interview someone else in the room. A different person needs to answer each question.

   5. Reconvene and discuss. Ask group members…
      a. What did you learn about yourself?
      b. What did you learn about someone else?
      c. Which questions, if any, would you ask when first meeting someone? When you know someone well?

Activity handout and facilitator's information submitted by Sherrie L. Easton, LMSW, Valdosta, GA.
Sherrie conducts individual, family and group therapy for children ages 4 to 18. She works with a variety of issues including ADHD, sexual abuse, anxiety disorders, and works closely with school teachers and administrators. Sherrie enjoys the outdoors and loves to go camping with her family, likes arts and crafts, and is an animal foster parent, involved in her local humane society.

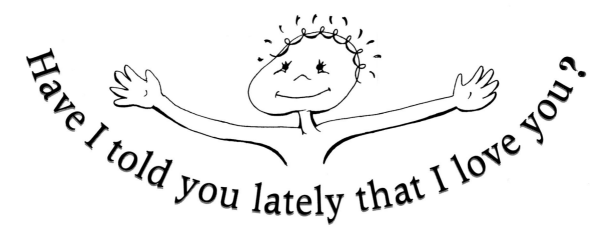

Have I told you lately that I love you?

Date: _____

Dear _____ ,

I just wanted to let you know how much you mean to me.

The thing I love most about you is _____
_____
_____.

Something that I do not tell you often enough is _____.

You have helped me in many ways, for example, _____
_____
_____
_____.

If I could wish one thing for you, it would be _____
_____
_____.

When I think of you I feel _____
_____.

Thank you for being such an important part of my life. You are very special to me.

Love,

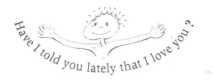

Have I told you lately that I love you?

I. PURPOSE:

To increase the ability to communicate personal, positive feelings with those close to us.

To increase awareness of the importance of communicating feelings with those close to us.

II. GENERAL COMMENTS:

Many people have caregivers or people whom they depend upon a great deal for help or support. For various reasons, many have difficulty expressing appreciation to this important person. We often think others know how we feel, and sometimes we assume this rather than go out of our way to express our feelings to those closest to us. This activity provides the opportunity for a detailed expression of positive feelings.

III. POSSIBLE ACTIVITIES:

A. 1. Begin with a general discussion about communication skills and the importance of being able to communicate effectively.

2. Ask each group participant to think of the most supportive person involved in his or her life at this time. If the participant is unable to identify only one person, more handouts may be given to that person if desired.

3. Ask each group member to recall the last time s/he articulated his/her feelings to this person and really expressed appreciation for this person's role in his/her life.

4. Distribute handouts and pens and review with the group.

5. Instruct group members to complete the handout, being as specific as possible when writing responses.

6. Ask how it felt to be able to communicate positive feelings to a loved one. Explore this in discussion.

7. Ask if anyone would like to share what s/he wrote with the loved one.

8. Provide envelopes for those who would like to give or send the letter to the identified loved one.

9. Discuss how the loved one may feel upon receiving the letter and how this may open doors to communication.

B. 1. Discuss the concept that when we are not feeling our best, it is possible that we don't show our appreciation or gratitude to those who are helping us. Ask for feedback or personal examples if group members are able to share.

2. Distribute handouts and pens.

3. Give group ten minutes to complete, encouraging them to put a personal postscript (P.S.) at the bottom if there are still unsaid thoughts.

4. Divide group into pairs allowing each pair to read and share letters with their partners.

5. Reconvene and discuss how important open lines of communication are. Discuss or give examples how showing and expressing appreciation or other positive feelings builds relationships, whereas not expressing positive feelings might distance people.

6. Discuss ways of expressing positive emotions in the future: sending cards, small notes on refrigerator, lunch box, etc.

Activity handout and facilitator's information submitted by Sandra Netto-Marceau, MSW, LICSW, Merrimack, NH.
Sandra's job includes group psychotherapy with elders, family support and education and individual assessments.
Her leisure interests include cooking, baking, reading, and spending time with her daughter.

The Talking Body

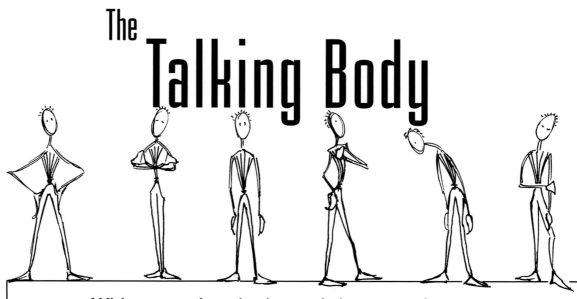

Without even knowing it, people interpret what we are saying through our body language. Are you telling others something you do not really mean by the use of your body?

Match the following body language characteristics with what you believe it is expressing. After you are completed, the answers will be discussed.

Use the emotion words at the bottom of the page
(you can use an emotions word more than once) or add your own.

Body Language	Emotion Expressed
Crossed arms	_____
Biting fingernails	_____
Wringing hands	_____
Rubbing back of neck	_____
Sitting on edge of chair	_____
Chewing pen	_____
Leaning closer	_____
Smiling	_____
Hand on face	_____
Leaning away	_____
Shoulders back	_____
Chin up	_____

ANGER ANXIOUS AVOIDING	BOREDOM CONFIDENT	COOPERATIVE DEFENSIVE EMBARRASSMENT	FRUSTRATION INTERESTED	OPENNESS PROUD TIRED

It is important to be aware of what people are telling us through their body language, and we should recognize that we are also communicating with our 'Talking Body.'

The Talking Body

I. PURPOSE:

To increase communication skills through the understanding and practice of various nonverbal communication cues.

II. GENERAL COMMENTS:

Effective communication depends on verbal communication with such variables as word choices, voice volume and tone, and nonverbal communication focusing on nuances of unspoken language. These nonverbal cues might be unnoticed by some and ignored by others, and possibly thought of as subtle, meaningless actions.

III. POSSIBLE ACTIVITIES:

A. 1. Discuss meaning of body language.
   2. Distribute handouts and pens.
   3. Define and explain any new or challenging vocabulary.
   4. Instruct individuals to complete the handout.
   5. Discuss the responses, modifying any answers that were incorrect.
   6. Discuss positive and negative messages that are sent out by nonverbal communication.
   7. Offer the following as charades, or make up some of your own, to demonstrate nonverbal body language:
      a. getting disappointing news in the mail
      b. getting excited by an invitation in the mail
      c. being surprised at your surprise birthday party
      d. feeling frustrated with your bills
   8. Process benefits of the understanding and use of nonverbal messages.

B. 1. Discuss meaning of body language.
   2. Brainstorm as a group, different ways of using body language to communicate emotions.
   3. Distribute handouts and pens. Discuss any new or challenging vocabulary.
   4. Instruct group to divide into pairs and act out each of the different body postures listed and have the other person write the emotion s/he believes is expressed. Then, instruct the partner to do the same.
   5. Allow five minutes for partners to review and compare answers with each other.
   6. Reconvene and discuss variety of correct responses.
   7. Process the benefits of understanding and using nonverbal messages in communicating with others.

Activity handout and facilitator's information submitted by Nicole Bilodeau Shea, MOT, OTR/L, Tampa, FL.
Nicole is working at a hospital in acute and outpatient care.
Her leisure interests are rollerblading, reading and playing with her dogs and cats!

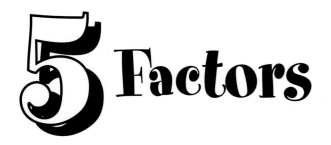# 5 Factors

5 factors have been identified that increase vulnerability to depression.

Which one(s) do you feel is a factor in your life?
In what ways can you improve these factors?

1 ☐ Having low self-esteem.

_____
_____
_____
_____

2 ☐ Constant negative thinking.

_____
_____
_____
_____

3 ☐ Inability to express oneself.

_____
_____
_____
_____

4 ☐ No social support network.

_____
_____
_____
_____

5 ☐ Poor stress management.

_____
_____
_____
_____

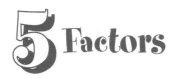

5 Factors

I. PURPOSE:

To increase awareness of factors that may increase the likelihood or contribute to depression.

II. GENERAL COMMENTS:

Certain protective factors have been found to decrease vulnerability to stress. Once recognized, steps can be taken to improve coping skills in that area.

III. POSSIBLE ACTIVITIES:

A. 1. Distribute pens / pencils and handouts.
   2. Ask each person to put a check in the box beside the factor that has had a large impact on their life.
   3. Give group members five to ten minutes to write three ways to improve the checked area.
   4. Share aloud as a group, supporting group members for insights expressed.

B. 1. Divide group into five subgroups.
   2. Give each sub-group a pen and a blank sheet of paper.
   3. Assign each subgroup a topic: having low self-esteem, constant negative thinking, inability to express oneself, no social support network, poor stress management.
   4. Ask each subgroup to write down at least three ways this factor might contribute to depression and then three ways to improve upon it.
   5. Allow each group to share results.
   6. Now, distribute one handout to each person.

Activity handout and facilitator's information submitted by Kathy L. Parker, COTA/L, Urbana, IL.
Kathy provides 1:1 and group therapy for adult and geriatric psychiatric inpatients. Treatment is directed towards restoring and maintaining optimal levels of psychosocial functioning by using a variety of tools and media, including the Life Management Skills series. She enjoys the computer, camping, gardening, sewing, reading, games and crafting – and most of all, being with family and friends.

Breaking Down Barriers

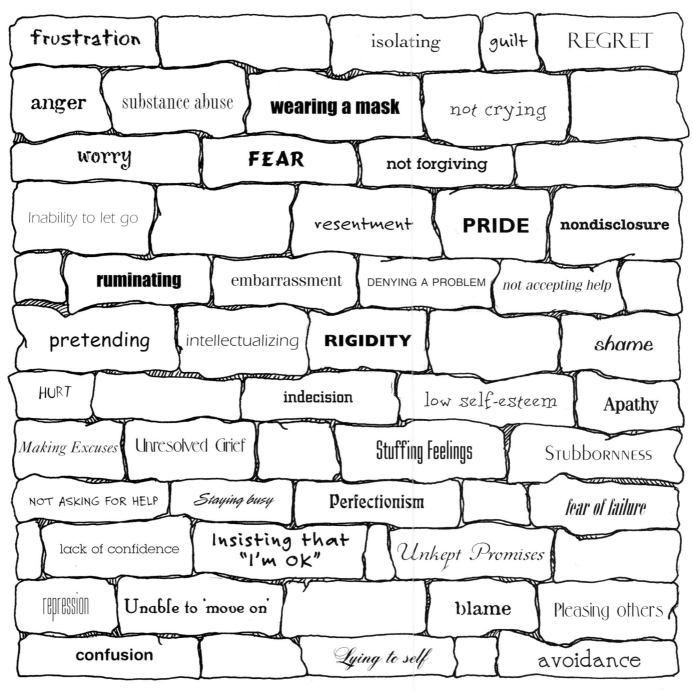

frustration   isolating   guilt   REGRET

anger   substance abuse   **wearing a mask**   not crying

worry   **FEAR**   not forgiving

Inability to let go   resentment   **PRIDE**   **nondisclosure**

ruminating   embarrassment   DENYING A PROBLEM   *not accepting help*

pretending   intellectualizing   **RIGIDITY**   shame

HURT   **indecision**   low self-esteem   **Apathy**

Making Excuses   Unresolved Grief   **Stuffing Feelings**   Stubbornness

NOT ASKING FOR HELP   *Staying busy*   Perfectionism   *fear of failure*

lack of confidence   Insisting that "I'm OK"   *Unkept Promises*

repression   Unable to 'move on'   blame   Pleasing others

confusion   *Lying to self*   avoidance

INSIGHTS:

_____ is my biggest barrier(s).

It prevents me from _____ .

I can confront this barrier by _____ .

Breaking Down Barriers

I. PURPOSE:

To identify and explore barriers to wellness or recovery.

II. GENERAL COMMENTS:

Barriers can be visually represented as bricks in a wall. Individuals working on a specific problem often-times speak of 'getting over' the problem versus 'getting through it.' We can dig under, climb over or go around the problem (the wall), but true resolution comes about by breaking the barrier, first by identifying and then by confronting it! This activity provides an opportunity to give this barrier(s) a name and work on assuming personal responsibility.

III. POSSIBLE ACTIVITIES:

A. 1. Ask each group member where s/he would like to 'be' (emotionally, geographically, spiritually, professionally, etc.). List these on flipchart. Answers may look like this:
- a. Not feeling so depressed
- b. Able to visit my family in another state
- c. Not feeling so angry
- d. Get a job

2. Then ask what each person's focus is, his/her goals towards wellness or recovery and what motivates him/her. Using a wipe-off board or flipchart, write responses, small enough for the facilitator to see.

3. Create a physical barrier of some sort (a large sheet of paper or other covering, as long as it is large enough to hide the written responses.)

4. Remind group members that although a barrier exists between them and their identified 'focus,' their 'focus' remains on the board. (Group leader can partially remove barrier to show participants, then return it to hide their responses).

5. Distribute handouts, markers/highlighters and pens.

6. Ask group members to identify and color a possible barrier(s) that they think (or believe) is obstructing their view, preventing progress or getting them to where they want to 'be.' Encourage group members to write unidentified personal barriers in the empty bricks.

7. Discuss how these barriers prevent progress.

8. Discuss ways on how to remove their barriers. As each participant considers and talks about a possible resolution, group leader can remove the physical barrier little by little until each group member's 'focus' is restored on the original board or flipchart.

9. Remind participants that although barriers to wellness/recovery present themselves from time to time, this does not mean a person's original focus is lost.

10. Give group five minutes to complete bottom section. Share.

B. 1. Explain concept of group by reviewing GENERAL COMMENTS.

2. Ask each group member where s/he would like to 'be' (emotionally, geographically, spiritually, professionally, etc.). List these on flipchart. Answers may look like this:
- a. Not feeling so depressed
- b. Able to visit my family in another state
- c. Not feeling so angry
- d. Get a job

3. Then ask what each person's 'focus' is and his/her goals towards wellness or recovery. List these also.

4. Distribute handouts and pens.

5. Choose volunteers to portray how this works. Participate as needed to demonstrate the concept. Volunteer #1 identifies a 'focus' from the flipchart that is also a direction of his/hers, e.g., go to a support group on a weekly basis. Then s/he stands about six feet from the flipchart and faces it.

6. Other group members review their handouts and volunteer to help by saying aloud, one at a time, what MIGHT BE a barrier. Avoidance? Not accepting help? Anger? Low self-esteem? Then the first volunteer should sit down and allow another volunteer to stand and let group members assist them until they agree with the barrier/obstacle.

7. Repeat this for the integrative experience as many times as group wants/needs.

8. Generate group discussion, encouraging group members to explore reasons for, and consequences of, each participant's barrier, along with how it is preventing them from reaching their 'focus' or goal.

9. Discuss ways on how to remove the barrier(s).

10. Give group five minutes to complete bottom section.

11. Divide group into pairs and allow a few minutes to share insights.

Activity handout and facilitator's information submitted by Mark S. Macko, MEd Psychology in Education, BS Psychology, AAS Graphic Art & Design, Sarasota, FL. Mark is a rehabilitation counselor who counsels and case manages disabled veterans in vocational rehabilitation. His leisure interests are creative writing, 12-string guitar, CD's and music videos.

FISHING TO FEEL GOOD

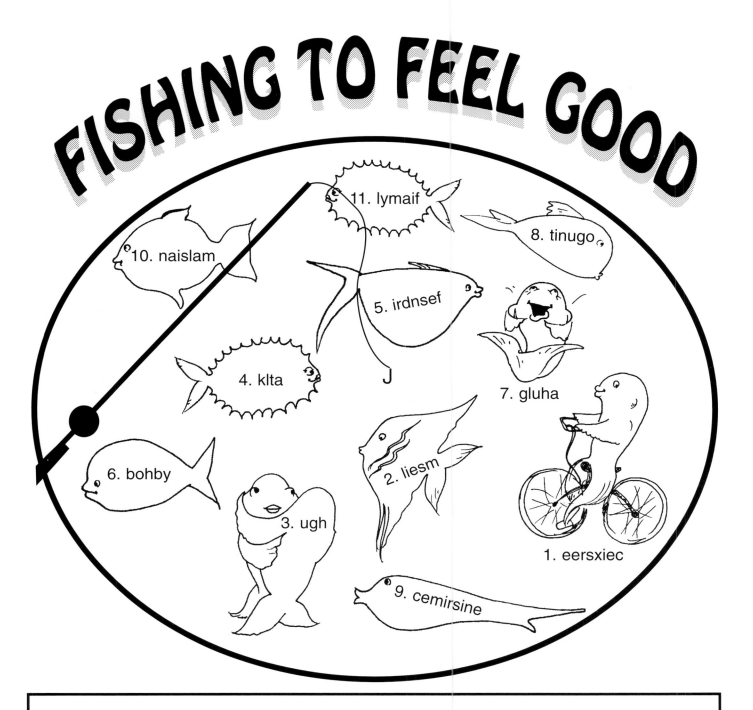

11. lymaif
8. tinugo
10. naislam
5. irdnsef
4. klta
7. gluha
J
6. bohby
2. liesm
3. ugh
1. eersxiec
9. cemirsine

DIRECTIONS:

Use the following space to list the scrambled words as well as other things that make you feel better about yourself, stronger, or better able to cope.

_____

_____

Name one thing you can do to make yourself feel better today and describe how to make it happen (or how you can make it happen)!

_____

_____

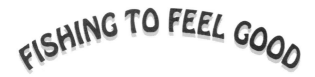
FISHING TO FEEL GOOD

I. PURPOSE:

To increase the ability to cope with daily stressors and the symptoms of an illness.

II. GENERAL COMMENTS:

Many times when people are symptomatic, they lose touch with all of the things they loved doing and become isolated, lethargic and (further) depressed. This activity is designed to remind people about previous coping skills or open them up to the possibilities of new ones.

III. POSSIBLE ACTIVITIES:

A. 1. Explain purpose of session using General Comments above as a guide.

2. Cut the 11 'fish' apart. Write corresponding unscrambled words on each and put in basket.

3. Ask group members to choose a 'fish' and have others guess what it is. They can act out as in charades, with or without words, or draw clues on board.

4. Distribute handouts and pencils. Instruct group members to complete.

5. Review correct answers and share those not listed on handout.

6. Discuss obstacles to using these coping skills when symptomatic, and problem solve ways of continuing to use them when feeling well and when symptoms occur. Offer examples such as having supports, setting goals, having enough activities from which to choose.

7. Process by asking group members to share one goal associated with today's group.

B. 1. Discuss the purpose of the activity.

2. Instruct group members to share one activity that helps them to 'feel good.'

3. Distribute handouts and pencils.

4. Give group members 15 minutes to list unscrambled words in addition to other things that make them feel good. Remind group that only safe, healthy choices are to be listed.

5. Offer correct answers. Ask for individual's input for things NOT listed and write on flipchart.

6. Discuss if/when participants last did some of these activities and assist the group members in developing realistic goals for actually using coping skills after session.

7. Discuss what they have gained from this activity and how it reflects on intended purpose.

ANSWER KEY:

1. exercise   2. smile   3. hug   4. talk   5. friends   6. hobby
7. laugh   8. outing   9. reminisce   10. animals   11. family

---

Activity handout and facilitator's information submitted by Paul D. Zavala, MOT, Orlando, FL.
As a Master of Occupational Therapy, Paul provides hand therapy services in an outpatient rehab center.
His leisure activities include fishing with his family and wife, Stephanie, as well as playing tennis and basketball with his friends.

Feelings and their
TRIGGERS

It is important to be aware of how we are feeling and why we feel the way we do.
Below, write five different feelings you have experienced, one in each circle.
Then write triggers to those feelings on the lines of the arrows.

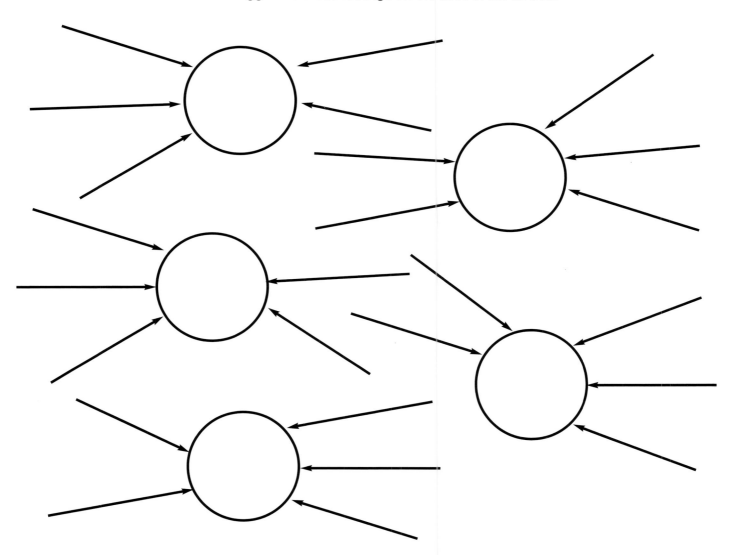

Think about what triggers you have control over.
What changes can you make to experience comfortable feelings more, and uncomfortable feelings less?

_____

_____

_____

_____

Feelings *and their* TRIGGERS

I. PURPOSE:

To develop an awareness of one's feelings and the triggers which evoke or provoke them.

To encourage the expression of one's feelings.

To promote behavioral changes which increase comfortable feelings and decrease uncomfortable feelings.

II. GENERAL COMMENTS:

Understanding what one is feeling is the first step in learning to express feelings and manage them. Understanding what triggers comfortable feelings can help one to increase the pursuit of behaviors, choices and activities – that lead to a more comfortable emotional state. Understanding what triggers uncomfortable feelings can help one to identify choices and situations that perhaps can be avoided or handled differently to lead to less distress.

III. POSSIBLE ACTIVITIES:

A. 1. Introduce topic including review of vocabulary (i.e. trigger).
   2. Ask each individual to identify one feeling s/he is currently experiencing. Then, ask for one trigger s/he thinks is contributing to that feeling.
   3. Distribute handouts and pens.
   4. Review instructions and ask individuals to complete handouts considering all feelings experienced recently.
   5. Share handouts as a group by either:
      a. asking one individual to share his/her entire handout at one time.
      b. asking individuals to choose/share only one feeling at a time until all participants have shared at least four or five feelings.
      c. exploring common feelings of the group. Have individuals share triggers to the common feelings, one feeling at a time, e.g., if several people list 'frustrated', have each individual with that feeling take a turn sharing his/her triggers to that feeling.
   6. Process common themes/triggers for comfortable feelings (e.g., accomplishing a goal, being respected) and discuss how much control individuals have over these triggers.
   7. Process common themes/triggers for uncomfortable feelings (e.g., failing at something, not being respected) and discuss how much control individuals have over these triggers.
   8. Close by asking each individual to identify at least one change s/he can make to better manage feelings.

B. 1. Use this handout as a homework assignment with inpatients or outpatients following a group dealing with feelings.
   2. Distribute a handout and pen to each participant and review vocabulary and directions.
   3. Instruct individuals to record feelings they experience during the day and the trigger(s).
      If s/he notices that same feeling again that afternoon or evening, instruct him/her to again record the trigger(s).
   4. Instruct individuals to return handout at the next session.
   5. Share handouts as a group by either:
      a. asking one individual to share his/her entire handout at one time.
      b. asking individuals to choose/share only one feeling at a time until all participants have shared at least four or five feelings.
      c. exploring common feelings of the group. Have individuals share triggers to the common feelings, one feeling at a time, e.g., if several people list 'frustrated', have each individual with that feeling take a turn sharing his/her triggers to that feeling.
   6. Process common themes/triggers for comfortable feelings (e.g., accomplishing a goal, being respected) and discuss how much control individuals have over these triggers.
   7. Process common themes/triggers for uncomfortable feelings (e.g., failing at something, not being respected) and discuss how much control individuals have over these triggers.
   8. Close by asking each individual to identify at least one change s/he can make to better manage feelings.

Activity handout and facilitator's information submitted by Tamara Cole, CTRS, Jeromesville, OH.
Tamara implements treatment for individuals on behavioral health and physical rehab units.
Her leisure interests include baking, crafts, outdoor adventures, movies and social time with friends/family.

If I could write a book ...

It would begin with ... _____

The easiest chapter would be ... _____

I would leave out the part about ... _____

My most difficult chapter would be ... _____

I would let _____ read it. (Specify: anyone, a few, no one)

I would / would not include information about all my family members.

My book would be more fact / more fiction. (circle)

The longest chapter would be ... _____

The shortest chapter would be ... _____

My book would be very long / very short. (circle)

A possible title for my book would be ... _____

I would dedicate my book to ... _____

I will / will not write a book about my life. (circle)

The last book I read about someone was ... _____

© 2002 Wellness Reproductions and Publishing, LLC 800 / 669-9208

If I could write
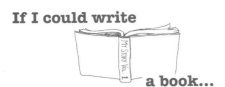
a book...

I. PURPOSE:
To increase emotional expression and disclosure.

II. GENERAL COMMENTS:
The ability to self-disclose has direct bearing on an individual's potential for recovery and self-discovery. Using incomplete sentence stems or starters, facilitates such disclosure, while incorporating an activity that condenses a person's life story.

III. POSSIBLE ACTIVITIES:

A. 1. Begin group by discussion of 'writing one's memoirs.' Remind each group member that although only a small percentage of people actually write a book about themselves – everyone's life story is interesting, unique and worth telling.

2. Distribute handouts and pens.

3. Encourage participants to complete the sentence stems (either verbally or written). Explain that there are no right or better responses, only different ones, since each person in the group is a special person with his/her story to tell.

4. Elicit responses from group members by :
   a) asking each sentence stem at a time for each person or
   b) having each participant respond to all of the sentence stems.

5. Expound on specific sentence stems. Explore reasons for what each group member would delete (if any), why a certain chapter would be more difficult to write, or the meaning behind the individual titles of books. Group facilitator could expound upon any sentence stem.

6. Begin group discussion about writing memoirs, providing benefits and values of doing so, e.g., "If it's not written down, it will be lost", "Each person has his/her own story to tell", "No one has a journey just like you", encouraging group members to get started!

B. 1. Begin group with discussion about journalizing. Talk about proposed benefits of journalizing, e.g., as a way to relieve tension, having a companion who is always available, an alternative means of emotional expression, a way of healing.

2. Distribute handouts and pens.

3. Encourage participants to complete the sentence stems (either verbally or written). Explain that there are no right or better responses, only different ones, since each person in the group is a special person with his/her story to tell.

4. Elicit responses from group members by:
   a) asking each sentence stem at a time for each person or
   b) having each participant respond to all of the sentence stems.

5. Expound on specific sentence stems. Explore reasons for what each group member would delete (if any), why a certain chapter would be more difficult to write, or the meaning behind the individual titles of books. Group facilitator could expound upon any sentence stem.

6. Begin group discussion about journalizing. Encourage comments and questions from participants. Determine who has kept a journal (or diary) in the past, why they stopped, who is considering keeping one again, or for the first time. Remind members that they do not have to tell their life story, only take 'one day at a time' to express their thoughts and emotions.

Activity handout and facilitator's information submitted by Mark S. Macko, MEd Psychology in Education, BS Psychology, AAS Graphic Art & Design, Sarasota, FL. Mark is a rehabilitation counselor who counsels and case manages disabled veterans in vocational rehabilitation. His leisure interests are creative writing, 12-string guitar, CD's and music videos.

The Emotions Balloon

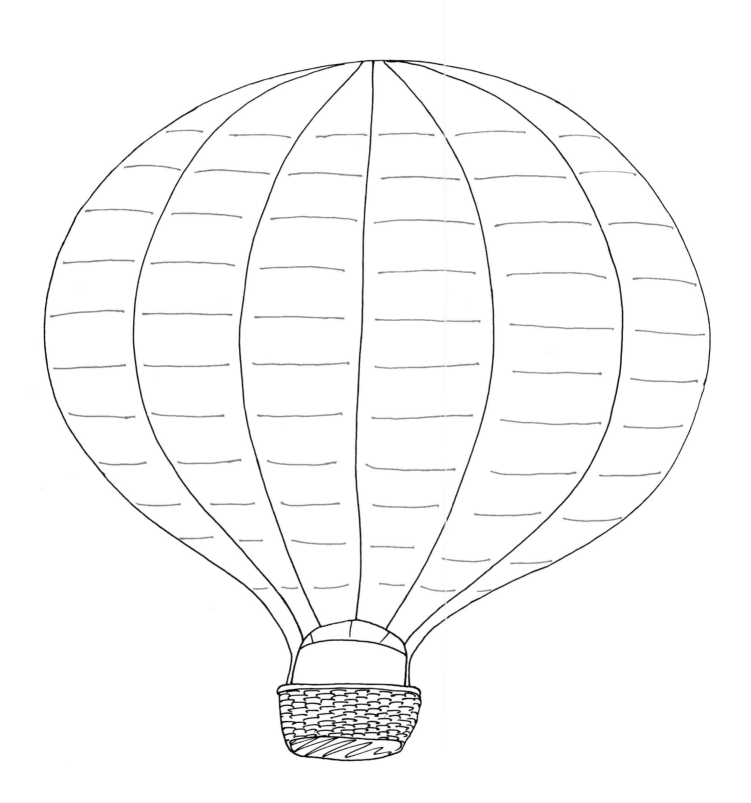

The Emotions Balloon

I. PURPOSE:
To understand one's level of emotions in response to real-life situations.

II. GENERAL COMMENTS:
Each person is created in a unique way and, as a result, will emotionally respond to situations differently. What produces a high level of emotion, such as anger, in one person – may produce very little in another. Taking the time and effort to think about our responses in a safe setting as well as explore the way we deal with them will give insight and opportunity for change.

III. POSSIBLE ACTIVITIES:

A. 1. Introduce the concept of having a 'threshold' for emotions and how using a balloon can depict this. A balloon can only hold a certain quantity of air before it will burst, just as a person who holds too much emotional energy may 'burst'.

2. Distribute handouts with pencils, markers or other coloring utensils.

3. Inform the group that you will be describing a series of real-life situations that may produce emotions in people. Examples might be:
> A surprise party is thrown in your honor.
> A tax refund arrives.
> Your teenager unexpectedly states s/he will be having a baby.
> Water damage happens to your home/apartment.
> Your significant other comes home two hours late with no explanation.

4. With each situation, ask group members to color in the balloon in relation to the amount of emotion they would experience in this situation.

5. After a series of situations are discussed (be careful not to come up with too many or every one's balloon will 'pop'!), ask the group members to show their balloons and discuss which situations caused them to color the most of the balloon.

6. Process by discussing ways of releasing some of the air from the balloon to guard against 'bursting'.

B. 1. Introduce the concept of having a 'threshold' for emotions and how using a balloon can depict this. A balloon can only hold a certain quantity of air before it will burst, just as a person who holds too much emotional energy may 'burst'.

2. Give each group member a balloon (make sure you always use new balloons for sanitary reasons) and inform them that you will be describing a series of real-life situations that may produce emotions in people. With each situation the group members are to think about how emotional this would make them and then to blow an amount of air into their balloon to represent their emotions.

3. After a series of situations are discussed (be careful not to come up with too many or every one's balloon will 'pop'!), ask the group members to display their balloons and discuss which situations caused the most air to go into their balloons.

4. Process by discussing the various ways in which emotions can be released by demonstrating the various ways in which air can be released from a balloon. For example, a full blow-up, a slow and whining release, short bursts, etc.

5. Distribute seven handouts to each group member (or correspond the number with the amount of days until you will meet with the group again). Ask them to record their real-life situations with colored-in spaces in their balloons. For example a small red blob has 'bill collector called' written in it, a large blue blob has 'dog ran away' written in it.

6. Reconvene next week to discuss.

Activity handout and facilitator's information submitted by Rick Germann, MA, LCPC, RPRP, Harwood Heights, IL.
Rick is the coordinator of daily operations for an outpatient psychiatric rehabilitation program. He also teaches undergraduate health and graduate counseling courses. Rick's leisure interests are anything outdoors! He is a field editor for an outdoors magazine and "when I'm not at work I'm usually fishing (with my wife, of course)."

GOAL con•nec•tion

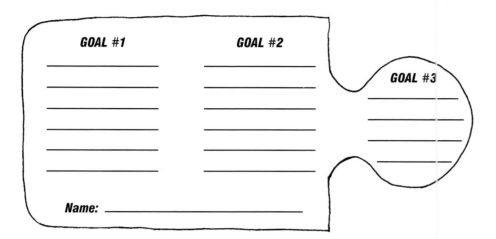

GOAL #1
_____
_____
_____
_____
_____
_____

GOAL #2
_____
_____
_____
_____

GOAL #3
_____
_____
_____

Name: _____

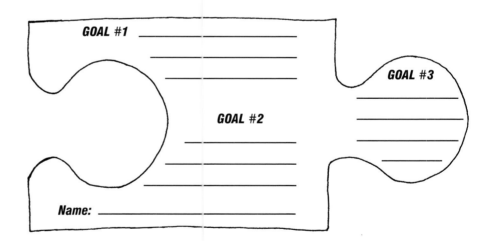

GOAL #1 _____
_____

GOAL #2
_____
_____
_____
_____

GOAL #3
_____
_____
_____

Name: _____

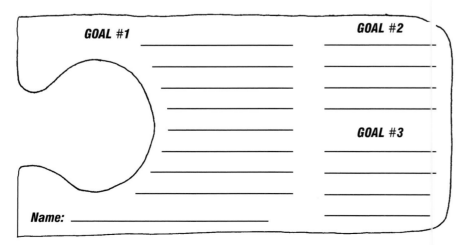

GOAL #1 _____
_____
_____

GOAL #2
_____
_____

GOAL #3
_____
_____
_____

Name: _____

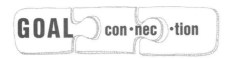

GOAL con·nec·tion

I. PURPOSE:

To motivate ourselves and each other by sharing personal goals.

To receive support and feedback about personal goals.

II. GENERAL COMMENTS:

Many goals are unmet due to lack of motivation. Making our goals known to others may give us the external motivation we need for goal attainment. In turn, one is more likely to accomplish goals while building and having support(s).

III. POSSIBLE ACTIVITIES:

A. 1. Photocopy handouts to be able to cut enough pieces so that each player will have one puzzle piece. Heavier colored paper works well.

2. Precut pieces to prepare for the group.

3. Introduce topic of goals. Facilitate discussion of personal accomplishments. Ask group members, "What are factors that get in the way of our goals?" and "What are factors that help us to achieve our goals?" Encourage feedback.

4. Distribute a puzzle piece to each group member.

5. Have individuals write three personal goals that they would like to achieve on the puzzle piece and their names. Set a target date for the group when all goals need to be accomplished.

6. Give group members approximately 20-30 minutes to complete their puzzle pieces and decorate them using markers, colored pencils, glitter, etc.

7. Ask group members to now complete their 3-piece puzzle by finding two other group members whose puzzle pieces fit into theirs. Ask the three-member group to share goals. The first person of each puzzle will be the motivator to the middle person. The middle person will motivate the last person; the last person will motivate the first person. Each person will end up being a motivator to a peer and being motivated by a different peer.

8. Hang the goal connection up in the room as a reminder to motivate and achieve goals.

9. Reconvene as a larger group and process. Reflect the message that, "Life is like a puzzle … you put it together one piece at a time. Together we will meet our goals piece by piece."

B. 1. Photocopy handouts so that each player will have one puzzle piece. Heavier colored paper works well.

2. Precut many of the first and middle pieces but only one of the last piece.

3. Explain the concept of realistic goal setting and how support and encouragement can be a motivating factor to achieving goals.

4. Distribute one playing piece to each group member.

5. Decide on realistic, short-term time span for goal (one or two weeks). Instruct group members to write their names and three goals on their puzzle piece, that they believe they can achieve within stated time frame. Give 20 minutes for this as well as decorating their goal piece with available art media such as craft stickers, markers, paint, etc.

6. Ask for one group member to stand up if they have a piece with a flat left side and a piece sticking out of it (the first piece). This person states his/her goals, hangs it up and then calls on someone with a piece that fits into his/hers (the middle piece).

7. Ask the next person to attach his/her piece to the first piece, to state his/her own goals, to restate the first person's goals (they can easily look at the previous persons goals on the puzzle piece) and state how s/he can support that person in meeting his/her goals.

8. Continue attaching puzzle pieces and sharing and supporting goals, until finally the last person shares. S/he will support the first person in meeting his/her goals.

9. Process by asking group members what value, if any, posting goals might have. Also, ask group members to be ready to discuss goal attainment in another session, after the time frame is over to see what was accomplished. Discuss what worked and what did not in getting goals met.

Activity handout and facilitator's information submitted by April Folsom, APPCM.

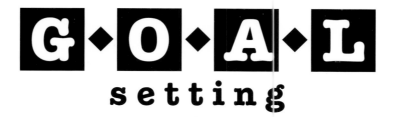

G•O•A•L
setting

THINK OF BASEBALL – the ultimate accomplishment and most challenging task is to hit a home run. However, a home run doesn't happen automatically.

First you must step up to home plate, and then three bases need to be conquered before the final achievement will be met.

With GOAL SETTING, defining your goal will be the first task.

Now, you must step up to home plate.

In baseball as a player runs from base to base, there are obstacles and challenges to overcome. The same applies to goal setting. Now, fill out the baseball diamond and plan out the steps, or bases, necessary to achieve your goal!

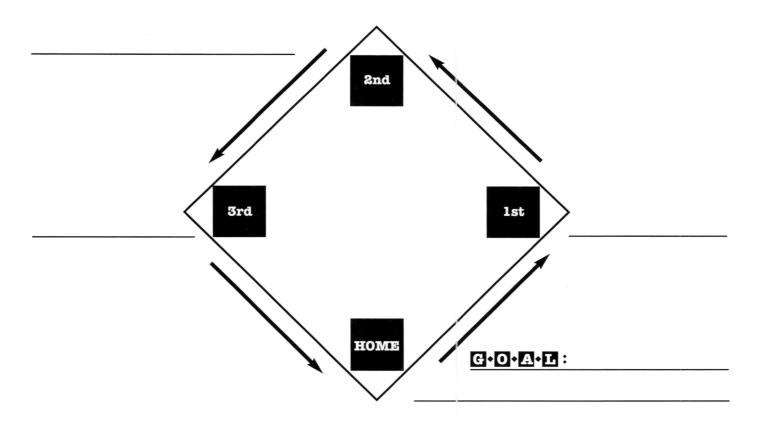

Possible Challenges & Obstacles	Ways to Overcome Them

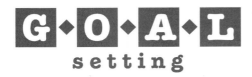

G·O·A·L
setting

I. PURPOSE:

To break down goals into manageable and achievable steps.

II. GENERAL COMMENTS:

All too often we have the tendency to set unrealistic goals. As a result, we become quickly discouraged when we are unable to achieve them. In the goal-setting process, there are steps we can follow to help ensure our success. These steps include setting a realistic goal, breaking down the goal into manageable steps and identifying potential roadblocks and ways to overcome them.

III. POSSIBLE ACTIVITIES:

A. 1. Distribute pens and handouts to each group member.

2. Read handout aloud.

3. Draw large baseball diamond on dry erase board with lines next to the bases as seen in the handout.

4. Elicit example from the group or use the following:
   Home plate = the goal itself - saving $100 in 6 months
   First base = make budget - getting help from Lucy, who is good with money
   Second base = figure out where money could be saved - decide on bank account
   Third base = know how much I need to save on a monthly basis (6 divided into 100)

5. Give group members ten minutes to complete top section of handout.

6. Share results and discuss.

7. Discuss possible challenges and obstacles in an open and honest atmosphere.

8. Allow group members to problem solve ways to overcome them.

9. Discuss benefits of this goal setting method.

B. 1. Explain basic concepts and steps in goal setting:
   a. setting a realistic goal
   b. breaking down the goal into manageable steps
   c. identifying potential roadblocks and ways to overcome them
   Offer examples as needed.

2. Distribute handouts and pens.

3. Divide group into triads. Allow fifteen minutes for small group work – facilitating group members listening to others goals, steps, roadblocks and ways to overcome them.

4. Reconvene and share.

5. Discuss benefits of receiving support and encouragement relative to goal setting.

6. Encourage the goal setters to report back to their small group regularly and the benefits.

Activity handout and facilitator's information submitted by Esterlee A. Molyneux, M.S., SSW, Logan, UT.
Esterlee is a program coordinator. She teaches parenting classes, provides in-home parenting skills, teaches an in-school sexual abuse curriculum, supervises children's anger management and social skills classes. Esterlee's leisure interests are scrapbooking, traveling, making crafts and spending time with family.

Hobby House

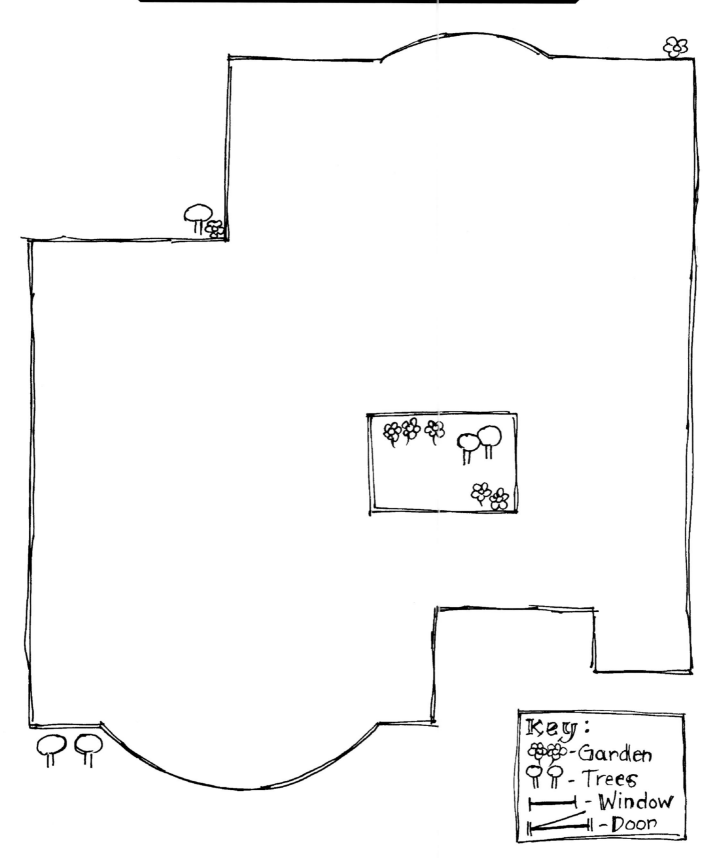

Key:
- 🌸 - Garden
- 🌳 - Trees
- ⊢⊣ - Window
- ⊢⧄⊣ - Door

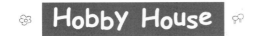
Hobby House

I. PURPOSE:

To identify favorite leisure activities.
To identify ways to incorporate favorite leisure activities in the home environment.

II. GENERAL COMMENTS:

Being creative about leisure activities may inspire some people to really think about what they enjoy doing in their leisure. Designing a 'Hobby House' is a fun way to explore leisure possibilities in one's life.

III. POSSIBLE ACTIVITIES:

A. 1. Ask group members to pretend they are the directors of a recreation center called 'Hobby House.' Brainstorm favorite leisure activities and list on flipchart.

2. Present to the group that they have the responsibility of designing 'Hobby House' with their personal leisure interests in mind. They are to be the architects . . . to design the rooms that represent their leisure interests. Pose the question, "What would make a perfect 'Hobby House' for you?"

3. Distribute scrap paper and pens/pencils.

4. Facilitate brainstorming session on rooms/areas they would like. Examples might include library, video arcade, music room, meditation room, aquarium, gym, nature center, scuba diving room but are not limited here. Stress creativity and personal expression! People can make notes about which rooms they might like in their own 'Hobby House.'

5. Distribute handouts.

6. Give group members time to create their own 'Hobby House' by drawing rooms and areas putting in details (recreation supplies, equipment, furniture, etc.) as desired.

7. Allow each group member a few minutes to present his/her own.

8. Facilitate insight by asking thought-provoking questions about what was learned and how this information can have meaning in incorporating favorite leisure activities into the home environment.

B. 1. Explain concept of being able to create one's personal leisure life based on interests, finances, talents, likes, etc.

2. Distribute handouts and markers, pens, pencils, etc. Explain that group members have the responsibility of designing a 'Hobby House' with their personal leisure interests in mind. They are to be the architects . . . to design rooms representing their leisure interests.

3. Give group members time to create their own 'Hobby House' by drawing rooms and areas putting in details as desired. Encourage group members to find separate or private areas of the room to work so that others do not see their work.

4. Collect all handouts after everyone is completed not allowing anyone to see each other's work.

5. Show each drawing one by one allowing the 'non-creators' to guess as to the originator.

6. Continue until all group members' 'Hobby Houses' have been identified.

7. Discuss that leisure is a personal expression of our selves.

8. For each activity mentioned (since they are preferred leisure activities for each person), ask how these activities can be incorporated into one's life more. For example, we know we can not have a library in our apartment, but how about a shelf for books, or a weekly trip to the library? We cannot have a greenhouse, but how about a few plants and planned trips to conservatories and greenhouses?

9. Brainstorm everyone's ideas, discuss and share possibilities for positive changes.

10. Ask group members to write three positive changes they can make in their leisure lives based on their 'Hobby House' creations and insight from the group discussion.

11. Follow up and evaluate the exercise and people's progress on positive changes identified.

Activity handout and facilitator's information submitted by Marty Golub, C.T.R.S., Rochester, NY.
Marty is a dependable friend of Wellness Reproductions & Publishing. He coordinates leisure service delivery in a Continuing Day Treatment Program for individuals with mental illness. He plans, leads and evaluates leisure groups. Marty enjoys bowling, football, crafts, traveling, volunteer activities, exercising, volleyball and visiting family in Chicago.

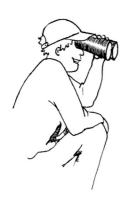

My Favorite Leisure

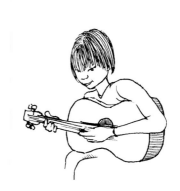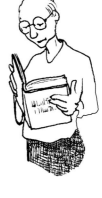

Scale
1 = like a lot
2 = like some
3 = really do not like

Category   **Favorite Activities in Category**

Category	Rating	Favorite Activities in Category
Physical Leisure	_____	_____
Social Leisure	_____	_____
Community Leisure	_____	_____
Creative Leisure	_____	_____
Spectator Leisure	_____	_____
Thinking Leisure	_____	_____
Cultural Leisure	_____	_____
Relaxing Leisure	_____	_____
Outdoor Leisure	_____	_____
Spiritual Leisure	_____	_____
Volunteer Leisure	_____	_____
Adventure Leisure	_____	_____
Solo Leisure	_____	_____
Home Leisure	_____	_____
Other	_____	_____
Other	_____	_____

What are the activities you would like to participate in more?

_____

_____

Do you have any ideas on how to get started?

_____

_____

What leisure activity category would you like to increase your participation?

_____

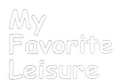
My
Favorite
Leisure

I. PURPOSE:

To explore the variety of leisure activities and experiences.
To identify personal favorite leisure activities.
To begin to establish leisure lifestyle goals.

II. GENERAL COMMENTS:

A thorough examination of leisure activities can lead to more meaningful leisure lifestyle goal formulation. This exercise can be an introductory session for a leisure education group. Group participants can work together to identify and brainstorm activities that can make their leisure lifestyles in particular more satisfying.

III. POSSIBLE ACTIVITIES:

A. 1. Distribute handouts and pencils.
   2. Explain purpose of activity.
   3. Explain the scale.
   4. Define each leisure activity category, e.g., Social Leisure is leisure that one participates in with others; Solo Leisure is leisure that one does alone; Creative Leisure is leisure that one creates something.
   5. Provide a few examples of each category, if needed, to assist group members to rate liking of each category. Even liking one activity in a category is OK for a "1" rating.
   6. Have group members rate each category for themselves.
   7. Brainstorm activities in each category. Write responses on dry erase board.
   8. After brainstorming each leisure category, have group members write their favorite leisure activities in each category. Stress that the amount of time spent on the activity is not important at this time, just that they like the activity. NOTE: Some activities may fall in more than one category and that's fine. Keep the brainstorming session fun and light.
   9. Next, have group members go through their lists of favorite leisure activities, circling the ones they would like to do more often.
   10. Discuss group member's findings and ways to begin the activities.
   11. Instruct group members to summarize thoughts in writing at the bottom of the sheet.
   12. Ask group members to identify activity categories and specific activities in which they want to increase participation. Using pages 14 (Goals) and 15 (One Step at a Time) from Life Management Skills I, have group members identify goals for their leisure lifestyles and steps to achieve these goals.
   13. Ask group members to discuss insights gained and process each other's goals. Follow up on people's progress.

B. 1. Prepare for group by:
      a. cutting one picture per category out of magazines of different leisure activities.
      b. writing the names of the 14 different leisure activities on the board.
   2. Show the pictures (not in any order) to group member and have group members identify the category to which the picture belongs.
   3. Distribute handouts and pens.
   4. Read together as a group, offering examples of each category.
   5. Explain scale and instruct group members to rate and identify the favorite leisure activities.
   6. Review findings.
   7. Pair group members and encourage them to problem solve bottom section together.
   8. Reconvene and process those last two questions.

Activity handout and facilitator's information submitted by Marty Golub, C.T.R.S., Rochester, NY.
Marty is a dependable friend of Wellness Reproductions & Publishing. He coordinates leisure service delivery in a Continuing Day Treatment Program for individuals with mental illness. He plans, leads and evaluates leisure groups. Marty enjoys bowling, football, crafts, traveling, volunteer activities, exercising, volleyball and visiting family in Chicago.

Realistic Monthly Budgeting

My paycheck for working 30 hours a week is $154.50.

This means I make _____ every month.

Bills I have to pay:

Rent - $250.00
Utilities - $85.50
Food - $100.00
Telephone - $45.65
Transportation - $35.00

In order to pay my monthly bills listed above,
I need to save the following amounts each week:

Rent: _____   Telephone: _____

Utilities: _____   Transportation: _____

Food: _____

---

1. I try to save $25.00 a month for emergency reasons.
   I need to put this much in my savings each week: _____

2. I have a balanced life so I include leisure / hobbies into my weekly activities.
   I spend about $10.00 each week on this. How much do I spend a month?
   _____

3. The total amount of money I spend on the bills listed above each month is:
   _____

4. Is there any money leftover in my monthly budget? If so, what will I do with it?
   _____

5. What type of miscellaneous things could come up in the month that I might
   not have included in my budget? How will I handle them?
   _____
   _____

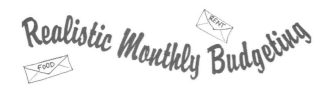

I. PURPOSE:
To learn, practice and enhance realistic budgeting for independent living skills.

II. GENERAL COMMENTS:
Many people have difficulty planning ahead with their money. Organizing a budget and preparing a monthly income can achieve a well-balanced lifestyle and prepares for necessities that otherwise could cause added stress. This practical tool takes a look at realistic expenses and asks thought-provoking questions to prompt independent living skills.

III. POSSIBLE ACTIVITIES:
A. 1. Introduce the activity by brainstorming all the expenses a person might incur, living in the community.
2. Discuss the difference between needs and wants.
3. Explain the importance of planning ahead for a balanced lifestyle, and to reduce stress.
4. Distribute handouts and pencils to group members.
5. Instruct group members to fill out the form individually, offering calculators if requested. Discuss results.
Correct responses are as follows:
   This means I make $618.00 every month.
   Rent - $62.50
   Utilities - $21.38
   Food - $25.00
   Telephone - $11.42
   Transportation - $8.75

   1. $6.25
   2. $40.00
   3. $516.15
   4. Add bills + savings + leisure = $581.15 leaving $36.85 left for emergencies, special occasions, etc.
   5. May include unexpected increases in bills, new medications or it could be related to family obligations. All other reasonable responses accepted.
6. Encourage note taking on handout and correcting answers if incorrect or give clean copy of handouts for correct responses.
7. Ask group members how this activity was beneficial and how they can use this information or skill in the future.

B. 1. Discuss obstacles in being a good money manager. Possible answers might include: "I don't have enough money to manage", "I don't have the energy or time", "I never learned that skill as a child."
2. Explain that money management is an important life skill that can be learned and practiced like other life skills and that even those people who lack wealth can still be wise about the money they do have.
3. Distribute handouts and pencils.
4. Allow group five to ten minutes to complete, offering calculators if needed.
5. Divide group into pairs to compare, and if needed, to correct results.
6. Review answers to make sure that everyone's answer is correct using A. 6 above as a guide.
7. Discuss question #5 and any issues that surfaced as a result from this activity.
8. Process by developing a plan with each individual to continue this process, asking "What is the next step for you in developing a realistic monthly budget?"

Activity handout and facilitator's information submitted by Courtney Behrens Bolduc, OTR/L, Goldsboro, NC.
Courtney works in a state psychiatric hospital in a dual diagnosis program, a day treatment program, and a community reintegration program for adults with mental illness – and is the treatment team facilitator. She coaches artistic roller skating, enjoys acting, dancing and choreography – and – writes poetry!

Resist Impulse Buying ... you CAN do it!

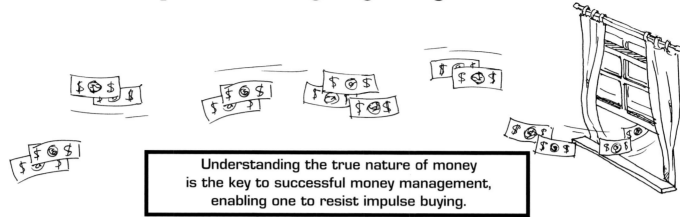

> Understanding the true nature of money
> is the key to successful money management,
> enabling one to resist impulse buying.

What money really is ...

1. **MONEY IS A TOOL.** When used well, money allows one to build, create, nurture and make possible what seemingly is impossible. When used poorly, money can divide, disrupt and destroy. Like any other tool, money must be used with good judgement.
2. **MONEY IS POWER.** The 'money tool' is very powerful and must be respected. Depending on its use, the power of money can either work for you or against you.
3. **MONEY IS VALUE.** Money is a means to an end. The use of money determines its value; money not used well has no value. Use it well!

Describe yourself as an impulse buyer: _____

_____

_____

Techniques to RESIST impulse buying:

1. Resist the urge to buy through your new understanding of money. Ask yourself these questions:
   A. Is buying this item now more valuable to me than saving my money for some other useful purpose in the future?
   B. Is this something I really NEED (or is it something I WANT)?
2. Understand that store displays and catalogues are set up to entice you to buy. Avoid the trap by again asking questions A. and B. above. Now, ask yourself, C. Is this what I originally came into the store for? Taking the time to think adds a delay that quickly diminishes the power of the impulse buy.
3. When faced with the impulse to buy, remember that you don't need everything. We are faced with hundreds of choices every time we enter a store; even a bargain is not a bargain if you don't need it. You need money for the things you truly need and truly value!
4. If you fall victim to the impulse buy, all is not lost. Give yourself credit for the effort to resist. Then offset the purchase by saving an amount of money to half the price of the purchase. Do this every time and put the money in a place where it is difficult for you to get it.
5. Your idea:

_____

_____

_____

> **Saving your money directly adds to your power by placing you in control.**
> **The more you do it, the easier it is. When you save money, you always have it for when you need it!**

Resist Impulse Buying... you CAN do it!

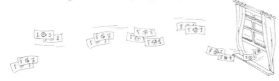

I. **PURPOSE:**
To understand the true nature of money and how to resist impulse buying.

II. **GENERAL COMMENTS:**
The nature of money must be fully understood before it can be successfully managed. Once this occurs, money then becomes a positive force of wellness and enrichment in life instead of a negative force of constant worry, stress and conflict. Impulse buying takes money away from other areas in our lives that might need it, often resulting in feelings of emptiness and guilt.

III. **POSSIBLE ACTIVITIES:**

A. 1. Distribute handouts and pencils.
   2. Review basic concepts at the top of handout, including the illustration, supporting disclosures regarding personal spending habits.
   3. Discuss common thoughts that set us up for impulse buying, for example, thoughts of – "I deserve this", "Maybe this will cheer me up", "I've had a hard week" and "I will never find this at such a great price in my whole life!"
   4. Divide group into pairs, to do the work at the bottom of handout. Assign each pair with numbers 1, 2, 3 or 4 as many times as needed. Give each pair five minutes to discuss their number's idea and to be able to present their understanding of their assigned idea. Ask them: "Could you see yourself using this technique? Why/why not?" Ask them to generate at least two techniques of their own to resist impulse buying.
   5. Facilitate group sharing of ideas and list all new techniques.
   6. Process by asking each participant to share an idea learned from this session.

B. 1. Set the stage for a buying exercise. Have impulse buying displayed as in a store. Place items in the front of an entryway in the group room, visually enticing participants. Impulse buying items may include candy, trinkets, magazines, soft drinks, gadgets, etc. Basic items such as bread, milk, juice, cereal, and eggs should be displayed with empty containers towards the back of the room. Write approximate prices on items. One or two persons are needed to act as cashiers, recording exactly what participants spend.
   2. Divide group into two teams. While one team is shopping, the other is observing. Teams will then reverse. If group is large, teams can assign one buyer, to represent the teams' choices.
   3. Each group member/team is given a total of $25 in play money to buy items in the store. Group members/teams are not required to spend all of their money. Set a realistic time limit.
   4. Instruct participants to spend their money on items for their household. Tell them that they are responsible for the grocery shopping and have only $25 in play money to buy items in the store.
   5. After cashier has recorded purchases, everyone can take a seat.
   6. Process by asking cashier to report on results of purchases. Next, discuss which items were impulse buying items and which were not.
   7. Discuss how impulse buying items are strategically displayed throughout the store. For example, stores purposely place items at the beginning and at the end of aisles, in open areas, checkout counters and at eye-level, to entice the shopper to buy on impulse.
   8. Distribute handouts and pens.
   9. Ask participants to complete blank lines and share as time allows.
   10. Process insights gained.

NOTE TO FACILITATOR:
On an ongoing basis, keep a file with collected ideas from the #5 on activity handout, (with permission from participants) and share with each future group.

Activity handout and facilitator's information submitted by Robert L. Vitelli, MS Public Administration, Skippack, PA. Robert develops and administers information technology contracts and business solutions to modernize federal agency operations. His leisure interests are investing, writing (watch for a fantasy novel!) and numismatics.

Are You Safe

from

Dawn to Dusk?

**Throughout the day we encounter many situations.
It is very important that we possess skills to keep us safe.**

The following events occur in everyday life.
Choose a topic below and give two safety considerations related to it.

Making meals	Cleaning apartment or house	Caring for the yard
Going out in public	Shopping (food, clothes, pharmacy)	Exercising (taking a walk, gardening, sports...)
Working with tools	Managing medication	Caring for others (babysitting, an elderly person)
Talking with strangers	Getting from one place to another, transportation	When going out of the home alone

Are You Safe
from
Dawn to Dusk?

I. PURPOSE:

To identify safety strategies to use in daily productive activities.

II. GENERAL COMMENTS:

At times, we go about our everyday lives without thinking seriously of possible problems which could result if we do not observe safety rules. It is useful to analyze everyday situations to determine what skills are necessary to remain safe at all times.

III. POSSIBLE ACTIVITIES:

A. 1. Distribute handouts and pens.

2. Have group discuss various topics and brainstorm to determine two safety considerations related to each, e.g., for making meals: watching stove, using mitts.

3. Write their suggestions on flipchart.

4. Discuss how important it is to be prepared for our current activity so as to reduce accidents to a minimum, e.g., have proper clothing, cooking supplies, training.

5. Process short and long-term importance of safety including ideas such as, to save a life, limb, time or money.

B. 1. Cut handout into 12 cards. Place cards in a basket.

2. Have each group member choose at least one card, read it aloud and give two safety considerations related to it. If someone chooses exercising, s/he might say "Stretch first when exercising and drink plenty of water."

3. Encourage group members to share experiences they or others have had, and the outcome of implementing or failing to implement safety techniques.

4. Discuss paramount importance of safety in our daily lives and the value that being safe and demonstrating safe choices might have for others in our lives.

Activity handout and facilitator's information submitted by Roberta J. Ott, COTA, M.Ed., Allentown, PA.
Roberta is a Therapeutic Activity Services Worker, providing programs to adult psychiatric patients, e.g., arts, crafts, music, coping skills and life skill development as well as community trips to prepare for discharge.
Her leisure interests are tole painting and reading.

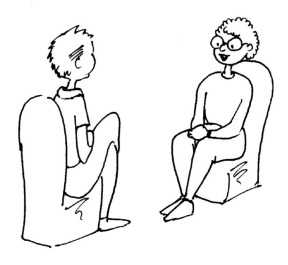

It's Your Interview!

There are no perfect questions or answers in a job interview, but practicing the job interview process will help you to feel comfortable, confident and prepared.

Write a job interview question on your 'Interviewer's Question' line. There is room for six responses from six different people. Have fun while learning other people's answers!

Interviewer's Question:_____
_____?

   Responses:

     1._____
     2._____
     3._____
     4._____
     5._____
     6._____

Interviewer's Question:_____
_____?

   Responses:

     1._____
     2._____
     3._____
     4._____
     5._____
     6._____

Interviewer's Question:_____
_____?

   Responses:

     1._____
     2._____
     3._____
     4._____
     5._____
     6._____

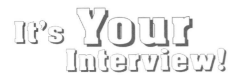
It's Your Interview!

I. PURPOSE:

To enhance knowledge of job interview questions, skills and techniques.

To instill confidence in ability to perform well in actual job interview situations.

II. GENERAL COMMENTS:

Many mental health clients have never successfully held a job and feel extreme anxiety at the thought of a job interview. This handout and activity will facilitate job interview questions and responses and will assist in reaching a comfort level regarding interviews.

III. POSSIBLE ACTIVITIES:

A. 1. Distribute handout and pencil to each group member.

2. Ask participants to put their initials on their handouts so they can be returned to them at the end of the activity.

3. Discuss the purpose of the activity and facilitate awareness about issues regarding job interviews. Openly discuss what's permitted to be asked in interviews and what's not.

4. Instruct participants to fill out the three 'Interviewer's Questions.'

5. Instruct the group members to pass the papers to the right. Ask each member to write a response to the 'Interviewer's Questions.' The originator of the 'Interviewer's Questions' should not receive his / her paper back until all responses are completed. (You might need to pass over the originator several times to accomplish this, depending on the size of your group.)

6. Share some of the responses and discuss the tougher questions and how to be prepared in the future.

7. Problem solve ways to be ready for a job interview. List on flipchart.

8. Ask group members to identify one thing they learned about interviewing skills that will assist them in the future.

B. 1. Write 'JOB INTERVIEW' on dry erase board.

2. With group input, make a list of questions that have been asked before or might be asked. Include questions that might be challenging for this specific group: e.g.,
   "Why is your work history so sporadic?"
   "Why are you just beginning work when you're 35?"
   "What are three of your strengths?"
   "What are three of your weaknesses?"

3. Distribute handouts and pencils.

4. Explain to the group that each is to write three 'Interviewer's Questions' on the handout.

5. Allow group time to interview six different people in the room. Each interviewee will answer three questions.

6. Reconvene and share what was learned. Discuss favorite answers.

7. Set up role-plays to demonstrate easy and difficult questions.

8. For closure, ask clients how this activity could help them with a real job interview.

Activity handout and facilitator's information submitted by Courtney B. Behrens, OTR/L, Goldsboro, NC.
Courtney works in a state psychiatric hospital in a dual diagnosis program, a day treatment program, and a community reintegration program for adults with mental illness – and is the treatment team facilitator. She coaches artistic roller skating, enjoys acting, dancing and choreography – and – writes poetry!

Highways to a Happier, Healthier Future!

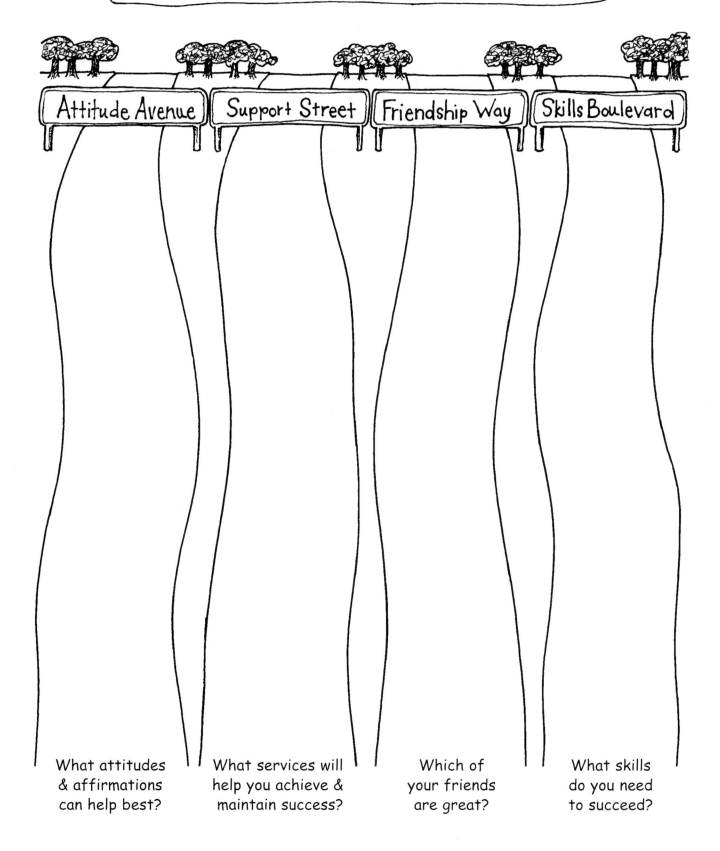

Attitude Avenue

Support Street

Friendship Way

Skills Boulevard

What attitudes & affirmations can help best?

What services will help you achieve & maintain success?

Which of your friends are great?

What skills do you need to succeed?

Highways to a Happier, Healthier Future!

I. PURPOSE:

To identify attitudes, services, people and skills one may need for recovery or a more successful and happy future.

II. GENERAL COMMENTS:

As people begin to look towards the future and maintain wellness it is best to be prepared. Many individuals might look less to treatment environments. An integral part of planning for wellness and recovery is to discover what is needed to achieve goals and access environments of choice.

III. POSSIBLE ACTIVITIES:

A. 1. Structure discussion on concerns for the future, hopes for the future and future goals. Discuss major life areas such as working, living environment, social/leisure life, education/learning, family, coping, moving on and accepting change.

2. List the benefits of planning for a happier future on a flipchart.

3. Distribute handouts and pens.

4. Explain concept of looking at attitudes, services, friends and skills in order to succeed at being and staying healthy. Work together as a group to complete each 'highway,' offering examples to illustrate.

5. Share results looking for differences and similarities. Ask group members if anything needs to be added to their 'streets' for a successful, happy future and/or recovery.

6. Process by asking group members what they learned about themselves from today's session.

B. 1. Distribute handouts and pens.

2. On the individual highways, ask people to write in what they feel is important to them for personal goal attainment and success in their future. Use prompts at the bottom of the page. Relate recovery goals if appropriate.

3. Allow for feedback and encouragement from group members while completing the handouts. Ask group members if anything needs to be added to their 'streets' for a successful, happy future and/or recovery.

4. Explain that the focus of each 'highway' should be "what needs to be present for one to succeed." For example, on 'Support Street', someone may say that as she progresses out of a daily treatment program and moves into the world of job training she may still require a case manager, a therapist and/or a job coach to succeed. Someone else may indicate, for example, that on 'Skills Boulevard', he will require budgeting and cooking skills to succeed in his own apartment as he moves out of a group home setting.

5. Process by asking one or more of the following questions:

   a. What attitudes need to be on your road to a happier future?
   b. What affirmations can help you face the future?
   c. What friends do you want in your future?
   d. What skills do you think you will need to ensure a happier future?
   e. How do you want others to behave towards you as you face your future and meet your future goals?
   f. What words of advice do you have for others as they face their futures?

Activity handout and facilitator's information submitted by Marty Golub, C.T.R.S., Rochester, NY.
Marty is a dependable friend of Wellness Reproductions & Publishing. He coordinates leisure service delivery in a Continuing Day Treatment Program for individuals with mental illness. He plans, leads and evaluates leisure groups. Marty enjoys bowling, football, crafts, traveling, volunteer activities, exercising, volleyball and visiting family in Chicago.

SELF-SABOTAGE

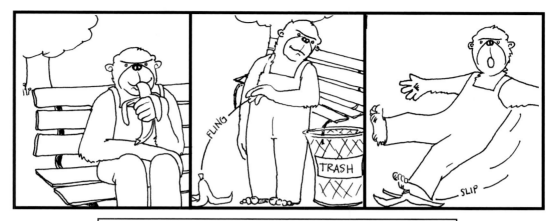

SABOTAGE:
-conscious or unconscious damage done to self by self
-self-defeating behaviors
-hampering one's own progress or recovery
-refusing to grow and change

WAYS OF SELF-SABOTAGING:

_____ **"Yes, but..."**
Using one excuse after another about why others' suggestions won't work for you.

_____ **"I'm different"**
Seeing yourself as different, worse, or more complicated than others and because of that, strategies that work for others just won't work for you.

_____ **Making the rounds**
Going from one person, helper or treatment to another, discounting what each says, looking for the answer you want to hear.

_____ **Stacking the evidence**
Only looking for evidence of how a treatment or suggestion may not work, while ignoring any evidence of how it does help.

_____ **Negative Comparisons**
Comparing yourself to others in a negative way.

_____ **"No way!"**
Refusing to consider new evidence, try new ideas or take any risks.

MY SABOTAGING

In which ways do I sabotage? _____

Why do I sabotage? _____

I will make the following changes: _____

_____

SELF-SABOTAGE

I. PURPOSE:

To develop awareness about how self-sabotaging behavior can inhibit recovery.
To develop a plan to stop self-sabotaging.

II. GENERAL COMMENTS:

Mental health practitioners will sometimes observe clients in the recovery process, acting in a manner which is counter-productive to themselves, despite all the new, helpful skills that have been taught. It can be extremely useful to facilitate a discussion with these individuals about how self-sabotage behaviors are a barrier to recovery. Since this can be a difficult issue for some clients to look at, it needs to be dealt with sensitively.

III. POSSIBLE ACTIVITIES:

A. 1. Introduce topic by asking participants to share the first word or phrase that comes to mind when they hear the term 'self-sabotage.' List responses on flipchart. See if the group can formulate a definition for the term, using their own words.
   2. Distribute handouts and pens. Compare the groups' definition with the ones on the handout.
   3. Invite participants to review the next section headed "Ways of Sabotaging" and to check off any items they recognize in themselves. Allow them to keep this information private if it feels sensitive, embarrassing or shaming to them.
   4. Facilitate a discussion about possible reasons people may self-sabotage. Ask them what insight they have into this phenomenon. Gently, and with sensitivity, review some or all of the following reasons for self-sabotage:
      a. fear of failure
      b. fear of the unknown
      c. comfort with what is familiar, despite the pain
      d. passive anger
      e. secondary gain(s)
   5. Have participants complete the remainder of the handout.
   6. Allow participants, if they wish, to share with the group their plan for stopping self-sabotage.

B. 1. Introduce / define the concept of self-sabotage. Normalize the concept to make it easier for participants to talk about by reminding them that, at times, we all engage in self-sabotage in different degrees and ways. Ask the group what impact self-sabotage has on recovery and healing.
   2. Distribute handouts and pens.
   3. Invite participants to complete the check-off portion of the handout, headed "Ways of Self-Sabotaging".
   4. Discuss possible reasons for sabotaging oneself. Refer to A.4. above.
   5. Divide group into sub-groups of three or four members.
   6. Encourage participants in sub-groups to discuss the last section of the handout. Focus on the statement "I will make the following change…" in order to help each other think of some ways to stop self-sabotage.
   7. Reconvene as a larger group and process by asking each participant to share one important insight they learned in the session.

Activity handout and facilitator's information submitted by Nancy Day, BScO.T. Reg (Ont), Markham, Ontario, Canada. Nancy has had 20 of her handouts published in the Life Management Skills series. She provides hospital-based occupational therapy services to clients experiencing mental health problems within a team-oriented program emphasizing group therapies. Nancy's leisure interests are quilting, reading, antiques and hiking.

Myths and FACTS about Mental Illness

If I feel like it, I can take more medications than prescribed. **Myth or Fact?** 1	Mental illness is always hereditary. **Myth or Fact?** 2	Taking medications is a cure for mental illness. **Myth or Fact?** 3
Denial is part of a mental illness. **Myth or Fact?** 4	Crack cocaine can bring on psychotic symptoms. **Myth or Fact?** 5	Family members and friends have important input about medications and symptom management. **Myth or Fact?** 6
Coming into the hospital again means you're a failure. **Myth or Fact?** 7	Mental illness is contagious. **Myth or Fact?** 8	If I'm depressed, beer will make me feel better. **Myth or Fact?** 9
Mental illness means you can not be productive. **Myth or Fact?** 10	Family and close friends don't need to be educated about symptoms when involved with someone with a mental illness. **Myth or Fact?** 11	You are not able to work at home or at a job if you have a mental illness. **Myth or Fact?** 12
Mental illness means you have no control over your life. **Myth or Fact?** 13	I can withdraw my medications without medical supervision. **Myth or Fact?** 14	Anti-anxiety medications can easily be taken for a lifetime. **Myth or Fact?** 15

Myths and FACTS about Mental Illness

I. PURPOSE:
To increase awareness of the FACTS about mental illness and dispel the MYTHS.

II. GENERAL COMMENTS:
Stigma, social climate and fear are all factors in how myths of mental illness have been perpetuated. Clients and families lack basic information and support. Creating an open, honest atmosphere enabling the realities of mental illness to be shared, can be empowering to all that participate.

III. POSSIBLE ACTIVITIES:
A. 1. Write on the board "KNOWLEDGE IS POWER!" Explain to the group that today's session will allow them to learn about the realities of mental illness.
   2. Distribute handouts and pens.
   3. Give group ten minutes to circle MYTH or FACT on the bottom of each of the 15 squares. Divide group into pairs, if this is helpful.
   4. Reconvene and discuss results. Explain answers if needed.
      (1) MYTH - Physicians need to be consulted prior to any change in medication taking.
      (2) MYTH - Mental illness MIGHT be hereditary, but not necessarily.
      (3) MYTH - There is no cure for mental illness. Medications, therapy and support are vital in managing one's illness, but at present, there is no cure.
      (4) FACT - Denial is a part of mental illness just as it would be a part of many other illnesses such as diabetes or cancer. Hopefully, as stigma decreases, people will be less fearful of having a mental illness and denial will be less severe.
      (5) FACT - Crack cocaine as well as many other street drugs can bring on psychotic symptoms.
      (6) FACT - Family members and friends can be great supports as they see things that perhaps the client does not see.
      (7) MYTH - Getting medical help is never viewed as being a failure.
      (8) MYTH - Mental illness is NOT contagious . . . even if others think it is!
      (9) MYTH - Alcohol is a depressant, it might feel like it's a temporary high, but it won't last.
      (10) MYTH - Being productive is defined individually and a mental illness does not prevent this important life value. People who have a serious mental illness may need to define for themselves what is productive and not let others define them.
      (11) MYTH - Remember...knowledge is power! Most relatives and friends can be supportive when included and educated.
      (12) MYTH - Being able to work at home or a job gives a sense of accomplishment and pride. Striving to do well in either of these roles is a great value whether it is as a volunteer, an employee, or keeping a clean and organized home or apartment.
      (13) MYTH - Individuals that manage a mental illness well, learn how to adapt and accept a situation. They have control to make healthy informed decisions and live in supportive living environments; symptoms do not mean that one has no control!
      (14) MYTH - Physicians need to be aware of any desire to go off medications so they can advise if agreed upon, how to do this correctly and safely.
      (15) MYTH - Anti-anxiety medications are, for the most part, for short-term use. They may be addictive. Alternate ways to manage anxiety need to be explored.
   5. Facilitate additional learning by giving each participant a blank handout to take home and play with a close relative.

B. 1. Photocopy handout on heavy paper and cut into 15 small cards.
   2. Explain that society has many fears and stigmas related to mental illness up to this point. There are many myths associated with mental illness. Now is an opportunity for change and it can begin here in this room today. Explain that at the end of the group all participants will know at least 15 MYTHS and FACTS associated with mental illness.
   3. Place the cards in the center of the table.
   4. Instruct a player to choose the top card and to guess whether the sentence on the card is a MYTH or FACT and to explain.
   5. Ask the group who agrees and who disagrees.
   6. Share the correct response and the explanation as indicated in A. 4. above.
   7. Continue until all 15 cards are used.
   8. Distribute handouts and pens.
   9. Allow participants to circle the correct response. Review.
   10. Ask group members to identify one significant person in their lives who might be interested, or benefit, in learning the information on this handout.

Actively Planning for Discharge

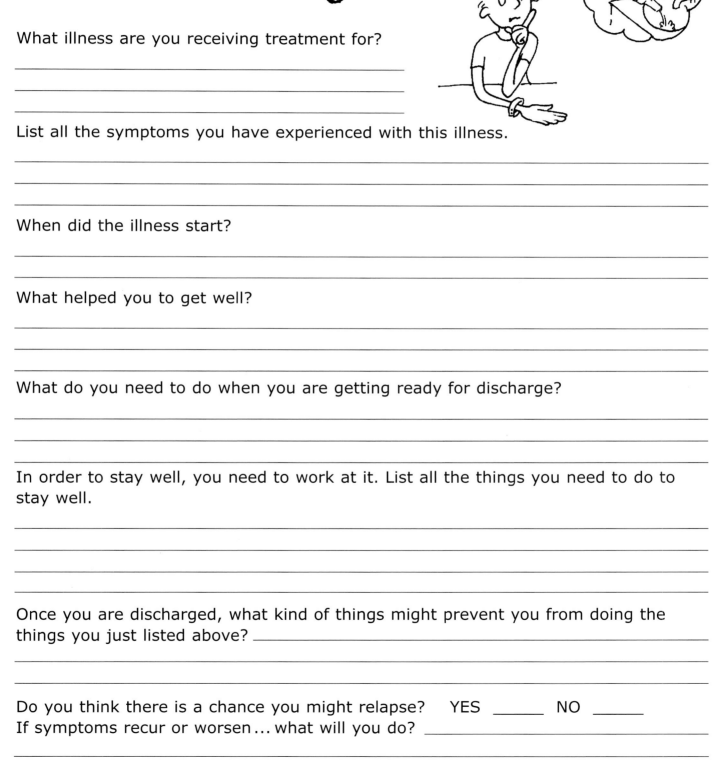

What illness are you receiving treatment for?

_____

_____

_____

List all the symptoms you have experienced with this illness.

_____

_____

_____

When did the illness start?

_____

_____

What helped you to get well?

_____

_____

_____

What do you need to do when you are getting ready for discharge?

_____

_____

_____

In order to stay well, you need to work at it. List all the things you need to do to stay well.

_____

_____

_____

_____

Once you are discharged, what kind of things might prevent you from doing the things you just listed above? _____

_____

_____

Do you think there is a chance you might relapse?   YES _____   NO _____
If symptoms recur or worsen ... what will you do? _____

_____

Actively Planning for Discharge

I. PURPOSE:

To increase the individual's awareness of his/her illness and potential for relapse.

To improve the participant's understanding of having to take an active role in preventing relapse and maintaining health.

II. GENERAL COMMENTS:

Understanding the illnesses which we have, is vitally important. We know that individuals are at significant risk for relapse if they have poor insight about their illness or a poor understanding of what they need to do to maintain wellness once they are treated. It is critical that individuals in treatment have a clear understanding of what they need to do in their recovery process as well as once they are discharged. Part of this process should involve identification of potential obstacles to health maintenance.

III. POSSIBLE ACTIVITIES:

A. 1. Discuss the importance of understanding illness, relapse prevention and discharge planning.
   2. Distribute handouts.
   3. Review the form discussing each question in detail prior to asking the group members to complete the question with their own responses. It is important to engage all group members in discussion, e.g., "What helped you get well?" Elicit responses about all that has been done to help them recover, e.g., medication, therapy, social support, structured schedule.
   4. After each question has been thoroughly reviewed, distribute pens/pencils.
   5. Ask group members to answer the question with their own response, giving consideration to what was just discussed. Emphasize that participants are to write a very personalized response, in their own words, as this will help them to retain the information.
   6. Have group members, who are willing, share their responses and read them to the group.
   7. After completing the form, ask each group member to take it home and consider sharing it with a loved one to engage support for health maintenance.

B. 1. Distribute handouts and pens/pencils. Draw attention to the graphic illustration. Elicit discussion of what "actively planning" means. Focus on the concept that when we take something seriously - we think about it, we spend time and energy on it and we actively plan for it. When we actively plan for something, we have a higher chance of succeeding because we thought of the whole picture - the beginnings, the possible problems, the ways to be successful, etc.
   2. Explain to group members that responses will be shared. Give group ten minutes to complete the handouts.
   3. Divide group into pairs. Give group members ten minutes to share responses.
   4. Reconvene into a larger group and give each individual a turn to share an interesting insight the other person shared or one way their partner shared s/he will do to stay well. Emphasize that staying well is also an active process, not a passive one.
   5. Elicit feedback from the group if this was or was not a helpful session and make sure that there are no further loose ends that need to be taken care of prior to discharge.

Activity handout and facilitator's information submitted by Betty A. Welch, Ph.D., Manchester, NH.
Betty provides clinical and administrative supervision of partial hospitalization unit and inpatient unit for geropsychiatric patients.
She provides direct clinical interventions with older adults, families and education to the community at large.
Betty loves spending time with her golden retriever, Casey, exercising, card making with rubber stamps and stenciling, hiking, enjoying precious time with family and friends, and creatively thinking about new ways to work with older adults.

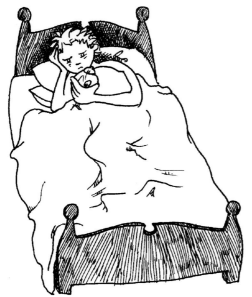

The "Just Right" Challenge

Healthy habits help to reduce stress. Yet sometimes we do too much or too little of a good thing. The key to coping with stress and symptoms of stress is to find the 'just right' level for you.

How well are you using the following coping strategies?
Place a ✓ in the box that best describes how you are doing.

	"too little"	"just right"	"too much"
Sleeping	☐	☐	☐
Exercise	☐	☐	☐
Medication	☐	☐	☐
Time Alone	☐	☐	☐
Social Supports	☐	☐	☐
Eating	☐	☐	☐
Thinking	☐	☐	☐
Distractions	☐	☐	☐

Which activities do you need for balance? _____

_____

How can you achieve this balance? _____

_____

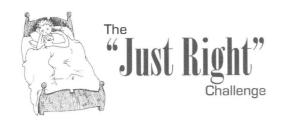

The "Just Right" Challenge

I. PURPOSE:

To identify which activities are being used as effective coping strategies.

To improve the overall balance and use of coping strategies for relapse prevention.

II. GENERAL COMMENTS:

Certain everyday activities can be both healthy and unhealthy, depending on how often they are used. It is beneficial for people to evaluate the balance of their participation in these activities to improve coping skills and the ability to prevent relapse.

III. POSSIBLE ACTIVITIES:

A. 1. Introduce concept of managing stress and symptoms as a way of coping with an illness and preventing a relapse.

2. Brainstorm a list of activities involved in maintaining a healthy lifestyle.

3. Discuss with group that these healthy activities can become unhealthy if done 'too little' or 'too much.' For example: The proper amount of sleep is essential for proper health. Too little sleep can cause decreased concentration, problem solving, energy, etc. Too much sleep leads to isolating behavior, lethargy, headaches, etc.

4. Distribute handouts and pens.

5. Instruct group members to rate how much they engage in each of the activities, considering how healthy the amount is for their lifestyle.

6. Ask each member to share results with group. Facilitate a discussion around emerging patterns.

7. Conclude by asking each member to identify one activity to work on balancing, and one strategy to achieve this balance.

B. 1. Write 'too much', 'just right', and 'too little' on dry erase board.

2. Give the following examples one-by-one: eating carrots, drinking water, watching TV. Emphasize that all the activities are OK to do, however it's how much we are doing them and how it fits in to what else we are doing that's important! Ask group members to raise hands when appropriate, e.g., "How many of you eat carrots too much? Just (the) right (amount)? Too little?" Tally group members responses and indicate the total numbers on dry erase board.

3. Explain to group members that one way to stay well is to self-monitor activity levels and to attempt a healthy balance of activities.

4. Distribute handouts and pens.

5. Ask group members to complete top portion of handout.

6. Invite group members to share results.

7. Ask group members to identify the outcomes of engaging in each activity 'too little', 'too much', and 'just right.'

8. Facilitate a discussion of how imbalance occurs in our lives and how this is related to relapse prevention.

9. Identify the top three activities in which the entire group would like to see a better balance.

10. For each activity, brainstorm strategies of how to achieve a balance.

11. Conclude by asking each member to identify one strategy s/he can use.

Activity handout and facilitator's information submitted by Enid Chung, Silver Spring, MD. and Beth Lucas, OTR/L, Quincy, MA. Enid worked as a mental health counselor in an adult psychiatric partial hospitalization program and also with inpatient psychiatric patients as an activities therapist. Beth Lucas is the Chief of a Psychiatric Rehabilitation Service. She manages occupational therapy services on three acute inpatient psychiatric units and provides direct OT services.

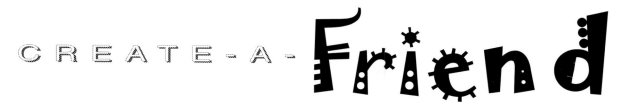

CREATE-A-Friend

Which characteristics do you find most important in a friend?

1. My friend should tell me everything s/he is feeling.

VERY IMPORTANT: Draw a ☺ for a head.

NOT IMPORTANT: Draw a △ for a head.

2. My friend should be a life-long learner.

VERY IMPORTANT: Draw a ⬭ for a body.

NOT IMPORTANT: Draw a ◇ for a body.

3. My friend should have a good sense of humor.

VERY IMPORTANT: Draw 〰〰 for arms.

NOT IMPORTANT: Draw ╱ ╲ for arms.

4. My friend should be good looking.

VERY IMPORTANT: Draw long brown hair.

NOT IMPORTANT: Draw short blue hair.

5. My friend should be willing to do anything for me, even if it's against the law.

VERY IMPORTANT: Draw red legs.

NOT IMPORTANT: Draw purple legs.

6. My friend should always do what is best for me, even if it may make me angry.

VERY IMPORTANT: Draw ✋ ✋ for hands.

NOT IMPORTANT: Draw 👃 👃 for hands.

7. My friend should be well liked by others.

VERY IMPORTANT: Draw 👣 👣 for feet.

NOT IMPORTANT: Draw ◯ ◯ for feet.

8. What else is important for you to have in a friend?

_____

_____

_____

My Friend

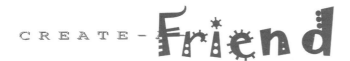

CREATE-A-Friend

I. PURPOSE:

To identify important qualities in a friendship.

II. GENERAL COMMENTS:

Many people are confused about what a true friend really is. Qualities and values that seem important during one time of our lives may not seem to be as important at other times. What is important to some people is not as important to others. It can be powerful to look at creating relationships based on our own current values and needs.

III. POSSIBLE ACTIVITIES:

A. 1. Distribute a copy of CREATE-A-FRIEND handout to each group member. Provide pencils and colored markers for the group.

2. Explain to the group that this activity is an opportunity to express what is important to each one of them as a friend. Tell them that there are no right or wrong answers. In addition, inform group members that they need not be artists to participate or benefit from this activity.

3. Instruct group members to read each item on handout and follow directions. For example, in question number 1, if it is important for the individual to have a friend who reveals all his/her feelings, the individual will draw a round head on his/her 'friend.' If this is not an important quality, a triangular head should be drawn. Depending on the level of the group, you may decide to read through each item and have members record their answers with appropriate drawing, or allow the group members to proceed individually.

4. Allow time for group members to compare their 'friends.' Ask the following questions:
    What is different about the friends we created? What is the same?
    What qualities do our friends share?
    What other qualities are important to have in a friend?
    What makes someone a true friend?

5. Discuss why or why not individuals feel certain qualities are important in a friend and what they learned from this fun activity.

B. 1. Lead a group discussion on qualities of a true friend.

2. Ask a group member to record these qualities on flipchart/dry erase board.

3. Have group members attempt to prioritize stated qualities. If a dispute arises about importance of a quality, encourage the group to reach a consensus through votes or discussions, acknowledging that each person has his/her own criteria for a true friend.

4. Distribute handouts and markers. Give group members five to ten minutes to complete handouts.

5. Offer opportunity for each group member to create new symbols for qualities and write and draw on board. Example: MY FRIEND SHOULD BE A GOOD LISTENER. Then draw large ears for very important; tiny ears for not important. After each person's turn, group members are to add those drawings to already drawn 'friend.'

6. Process by asking group members if they have true friends, if they believe they are good friends and how they might improve friendships.

Activity handout and facilitator's information submitted by Elana Blachman Markovitz, M.A., OTR/L, Forest Hills, NY.
Elana works in public schools with children experiencing developmental delays, physical disabilities and learning disabilities – to increase performance in the school environment. Areas of concentration include fine and gross motor skill acquisition and development, as well as use of assistive technology. She enjoys bowling and crossword puzzles.

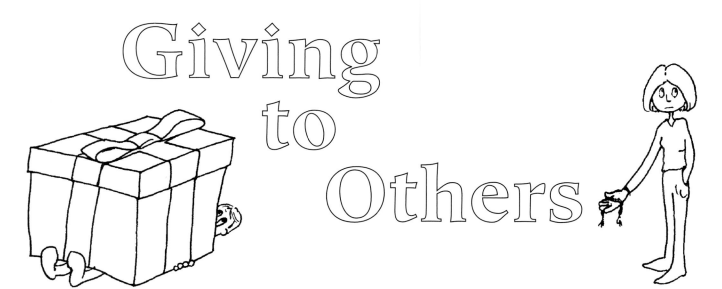

Giving to Others

DO I GIVE TOO MUCH? Yes __ No __ **If Yes ...** **Consequences to myself / others** overfunction for other(s) become drained feel resentful other _____	**DO I GIVE TOO LITTLE?** Yes __ No __ **If Yes ...** **Consequences to myself / others** lack of friends weak relationships feel guilty other _____

↔

IDEAS FOR WAYS TO GIVE LESS attend to my own needs encourage others to help themselves delegate accept help from others other _____ _____ _____	**IDEAS FOR WAYS TO GIVE MORE** smile more often make a compliment treat someone to coffee send a card or letter other _____ _____ _____

RELATIONSHIPS IN MY LIFE

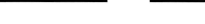

Name of Person   **What I Need To Change:**

1. _____   _____

2. _____   _____

3. _____   _____

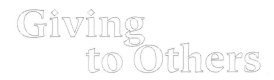

Giving to Others

I. PURPOSE:

To facilitate the understanding of appropriately giving to others.

II. GENERAL COMMENTS:

Individuals may have difficulty in relationships with either giving too much or too little. Those with severe mental health challenges may be isolated, have few relationships, and feel they have nothing to give and/or not know how to give. On the other hand some individuals have a poor sense of boundaries in relationships or have been taught to give endlessly, at the expense of their own mental health.

III. POSSIBLE ACTIVITIES:

A. 1. Introduce session by having participants, one at a time, turn to the person on their right and give him/her a dream trip (explanation of choice of trip optional). Briefly discuss feelings of giving and receiving this 'gift.'

2. Explain notion that individuals may have difficulties associated with giving – giving too much or giving too little. Ask for examples from group. Draw out possible reasons and insights behind the behaviors.

3. Distribute handouts and pens.

4. Instruct participants to complete top two boxes only. Discuss participants' own experiences with consequences.

5. Have group review next section and brainstorm additional suggestions for ways to give less and ways to give more.

6. Give time to complete last section of handout.

7. Conclude by having participants share one thing they plan to change in their behavior and the possible results they might see.

B. 1. Have group brainstorm benefits of giving to others. Facilitate some initial discussion on concept of appropriately giving to others versus giving too much or too little. If time allows, develop and tell brief fictional scenarios about 'Mrs. X and Mr. Z' who give too much or too little. Offer real-life observed consequences of these behaviors in your scenarios.

2. Ask participants to identify problems or successes they have experienced with giving appropriately or inappropriately. List on flipchart.

3. Distribute handouts and pens.

4. Allow ample time for group members to complete.

5. Conclude with a discussion in which each participant shares one thing they have learned during this session.

Activity handout and facilitator's information submitted by Nancy Day, BScO.T. Reg (Ont), Markham, Ontario, Canada. Nancy has had 20 of her handouts published in the Life Management Skills series. She provides hospital-based occupational therapy services to clients experiencing mental health problems within a team-oriented program emphasizing group therapies. Nancy's leisure interests are quilting, reading, antiques and hiking.

Excuses, excuses, excuses . . .

What kinds of things get in your way?
What do you tell yourself?

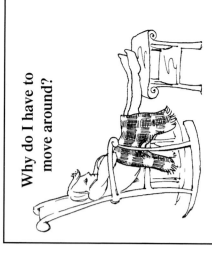

I've got nothing to wear.

My pajamas feel too good to take off.

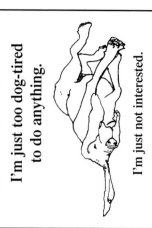

I can't handle it!

What will people say if they see me like this?

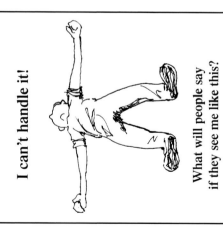

I'm just too dog-tired to do anything.

I'm just not interested.

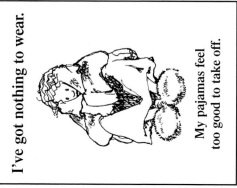

Why do I have to move around?

I'm just fine sitting here - it's not that important to be with people.

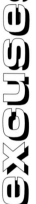

The excuses I tell myself most often are: _____

What I've been avoiding: _____

What can I do to change things?
I need to get 'unstuck' from that terrible position I find myself in. (I'm not 'lion'!)

My plan of action: _____

Excuses, excuses, excuses...

I. PURPOSE:

To increase personal responsibility by acknowledging the excuses that we sometimes use to avoid doing the things that need to be done.

II. GENERAL COMMENTS:

All of us have used excuses. Some of us are better at making up excuses than others. It is important to identify what kinds of things we are avoiding and how we utilize excuses to do so. It is equally important to identify a concrete plan of action to combat our procrastination or avoidance.

III. POSSIBLE ACTIVITIES:

A. 1. Distribute handouts and pens to each group member.

2. Ask different members to read aloud one of the excuses.

3. Encourage group members to talk about their own excuses and when they use them. This may require prompting of additional excuses. It is sometimes useful to inject humor as well, so that this is not perceived as threatening in any way!

4. Discuss procrastination and avoidance. Ask group members to generate a list of the types of activities people typically delay or avoid, e.g., doing their taxes, going to a social event where they don't know anyone, telling someone how they really feel.

5. Ask each group member to write on the handout what s/he typically avoids and the typical excuse.

6. Discuss with group members the importance of having a plan to actively combat procrastination and avoidance. Ask group members to write their responses and to make a personal commitment to change things.

7. If possible, check in with group members after an agreed-upon time period to see how they have progressed. If individuals have not followed their plan, review the excuses used in the intervening time period and develop more specific goals to address this in the future. Then, reevaluate.

B. 1. Begin group by introducing concept of looking at excuses as a way to address personal responsibility. Assign two group members to the following brief script or develop one of your own:

> Jonathan: *I'd love to see your place sometime, can I come over?*
> Maria: *Uh... No... not this week, I'm kind of busy.*
> Jonathan: *I didn't mean this week. How about next week or the week after?*
> Maria: *Well, my apartment is so hot in the summer... I don't have air-conditioning.*
> Jonathan: *I work during the day, evenings are nice and cool.*
> Maria: *Hmmm, Well...*

2. Discuss the following points: What could Maria be avoiding? What were her excuses? How can excuses pay a toll on relationships? How can excuses pay a toll on personal integrity? How can we tell when others are making excuses? How can we tell when we're making excuses?

3. Distribute handouts and pens, instructing participants to complete handouts except for the bottom plan of action section.

4. Discuss the drawbacks and consequences to making excuses in: activities of daily living, exercising, social outings/obligations, developing hobbies and leisure interests, writing letters, making phone calls, paying bills, going to see the doctor/dentist, etc.

5. Focus on plan of action by emphasizing that once awareness takes place, change is possible. Give group members ten minutes to complete.

6. Divide group into pairs and allow three to four minutes to share.

7. Keep group in pairs and have each partner report on their partner's plan of action.

8. Process by asking group members how insight gained in this group will assist them after they

Activity handout and facilitator's information submitted by Betty A. Welch, Ph.D., Manchester, NH.
Betty provides clinical and administrative supervision of partial hospitalization unit and inpatient unit for geropsychiatric patients. She provides direct clinical interventions with older adults, families and education to the community at large.
Betty loves spending time with her golden retriever, Casey, exercising, card making with rubber stamps and stenciling, hiking, enjoying precious time with family and friends, and creatively thinking about new ways to work with older adults.

Medication Management Strategies

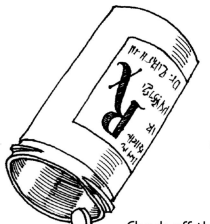

Managing medication well is an important part of recovery and relapse prevention. People typically need to try several strategies to find the ones that work for them.

Check off the strategies you have tried.
Underline the strategies that work for you.

- ◯ **Having medication with me in case I'm not at home.**
- ◯ **Putting my medication in a visible location.**
- ◯ **Reminding myself of what happens if I don't take my medications as prescribed.**
- ◯ **Someone reminding me to take my medication.**
- ◯ **Setting up my medication in a 1-week organizer.**
- ◯ **Setting up my medication daily.**
- ◯ **Leaving myself a note with medication times.**
- ◯ **Taking my medication with meals.**
- ◯ **Setting up an alarm clock.**
- ◯ **Taking my medication at bedtime.**
- ◯ **Other**_____
- ◯ **Other**_____

Are the strategies for your medication management working consistently?   Yes___ No___

If not, is there a strategy that you would like to try? Describe it: _____

MEDICATION MANAGEMENT STRATEGIES

I. PURPOSE:

To improve responsibility of medication management routines by exploring:
   a. difficulties related to adhering to these routines.
   b. a variety of effective strategies in achieving medication management routines.

II. GENERAL COMMENTS:

For some people, medication routines are critical in maintaining a healthy and functional lifestyle. Group support and problem solving can be effective in promoting and achieving an effective medication management routine.

III. POSSIBLE ACTIVITIES:

A. 1. Lead group discussion on the importance of medication routine. Discuss implications or consequences of not taking medications as prescribed.
   2. Distribute handouts and pens.
   3. Ask group members to complete.
   4. Encourage participants to share successful methods of adhering to medication routines.

B. 1. Lead group discussion on the importance of medication routine. Discuss implications or consequences of not taking medications as prescribed.
   2. Create ten index cards with one strategy on each.
   3. Place cards in a bag.
   4. Ask each group member to choose a card and discuss if this strategy would be beneficial for him or her. Proceed until all cards are used.
   5. Distribute handouts and ask group members to complete with support of significant others for next session.

Activity handout and facilitator's information submitted by Kathleen O'Neill, COTA/L, Hope, RI. Kathleen is an active member of an interdisciplinary team at a sub acute rehab facility. She provides direct treatment to patients, documents progress, performs home evaluations as well as participates in public relations, quality improvement and in-service programs. Kathleen's leisure interests are reading, cooking, sewing, swimming, hiking and camping.

Tools for Change

Tools **for Change** can be used to . . .

To make a significant change in my life, I need a _____ to _____.

To make a significant change in my life, I need a _____ to _____.

To make a significant change in my life, I need a _____ to _____.

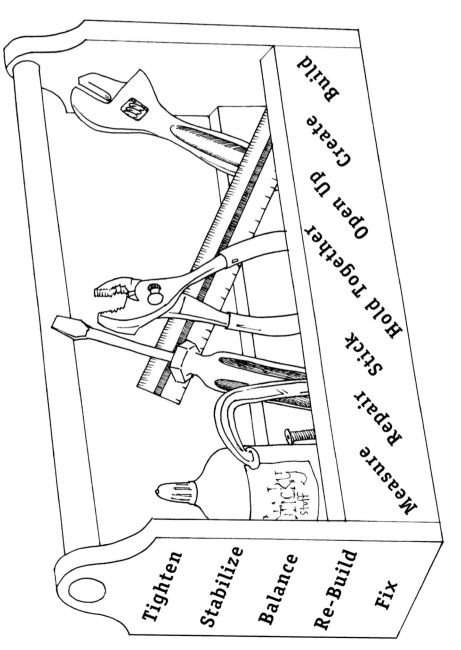

Measure
Repair
Stick
Hold Together
Open Up
Create
Build

Tighten
Stabilize
Balance
Re-Build
Fix

Tools For Change

can be used to . . .

I. PURPOSE:

To identify and learn the language needed to take responsibility for changes in our lives.

II. GENERAL COMMENTS:

People often resist taking responsibility for making choices that might cause change. This might be due to poor self-esteem, lack of personal resources, fear, etc. Taking responsibility for making changes includes looking at inner tools we have and the tools we need to make significant changes.

III. POSSIBLE ACTIVITIES:

A. 1. Facilitate discussion on purpose of 'tools.' Identify several things tools are used for, e.g., screwdrivers tighten things up, levels provide balance. Use actual tools for props if safe environment.

   2. Distribute handouts and pens.

   3. Encourage each member to choose three tools from the toolbox (or draw one/some of their own) and identify ways they may use these tools in their own life. Offer group members example if needed: "To make a significant change in my life, I need a _____(hammer) to _____ (pound into myself that I need to be accepting and not judgmental.)" "To make a significant change in my life, I need a _____ (bottle of glue) to _____ (stick to my commitments)." Ask group members to write own responses on the right side of the handout.

   4. Have members share their answers when completed.

   5. Facilitate supportive problem solving focusing on ways to obtain or use these tools to make significant changes.

B. 1. Facilitate discussion on taking responsibility to create changes in our own lives. Discuss changes people desire and obstacles to taking responsibility to make these changes.

   2. Use an example suggested from the group to illustrate concept or use the following: "A significant change someone wants to make is being more honest with a family member. Every time I'm honest I get in trouble."

   3. Discuss the 'tools' we need to begin to make changes. Ask someone in the group to find a tool that might assist with this and to explain. "The jar opener will help you open your mouth when you need to." "The level might keep you balanced and not going overboard in sharing everything you're thinking and not being hurtful."

   4. Distribute handouts and pens. Instruct group members to complete individually.

   5. Divide group into pairs and give a few minutes for sharing.

   6. Process with group members ways of finding or using these necessary tools for change.

Activity handout and facilitator's information submitted by Mary K. Tilden-Walker, B.S.W., L.S.W., Silver Lake, OH.
Mary is a school-based consultant, working with children and adolescents – assessments, short-term counseling, referrals forfollow-up services, group work and classroom presentations keep her busy!
Most of Mary's leisure time is spent with her children and involvement in their activities.

Group name: _____

Date: _____

Motivational Messages for _____

My group members gave this list of strengths, words of thanks, and messages of hope to me... with a guarantee of truth and honesty.

I will review this when I need support and motivation to stay on track:

_____
_____
_____
_____
_____
_____
_____
_____
_____
_____
_____
_____
_____
_____
_____

Two strengths that I have, and must use, to help me stay on track:

_____
_____
_____

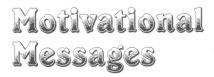

Motivational Messages

I. PURPOSE:

To provide written support and motivation between group members and provide a positive memory of the group experience.

II. GENERAL COMMENTS:

The power of positive feedback is energizing and touching, especially when it is given by people who have spent some meaningful time together, addressing an important issue. This exercise is suitable for use at the end of various types of groups such as self-esteem, weight loss, stress management and assertiveness. It is designed for the final session of a closed group series.

III. POSSIBLE ACTIVITIES:

A. 1. Distribute handouts and pens. (Clipboards if not seated at a table.)

    2. Instruct everyone to write their name in the space "Motivational Message for _____ " (Groups often appreciate when the group leader participates – so you might fill one out yourself.)

    3. Instruct individuals to write a message to each group member, and that the only rules are that the message must be:
   a. positive
   b. true

Otherwise the message can say anything. Examples include one word describing a strength you see in that person, a message thanking him/her for something s/he said that touched or helped you, or some change you have seen that person make.

    4. Ask the group to pass their papers to the person beside them. Provide time for everyone to write his or her messages. (It usually takes people longer for the first one or two.)

    5. Then, instruct group members to pass the handout to the next person, and allow time to write.

    6. Continue until the page is returned to its owner. Continue on the back if necessary.

    7. Before they read their own, ask participants to write a message to themselves in the space at the bottom of the page.

    8. Allow people to read their own.

    9. Invite people to respond to the group, if they want.

  10. Encourage participants to keep and review the messages. Explain it is a way of 'taking their group with them.'

B. 1. Discuss how motivational messages can serve to 'keep us on track'. Offer examples of messages of hope and discuss how this might feel to the recipient.

    2. Distribute handouts and pens.

    3. Divide group into pairs.

    4. Instruct individuals to write a message to his or her partner, and that the only rules are that the message must be:
   a. positive
   b. true

Otherwise the message can say anything. Examples include one word describing a strength you see in that person, a message thanking him/her for something s/he said that touched or helped you, or some change you have seen that person make.

    5. Instruct partners to return handout and give time for each to read either silently or aloud.

    6. Allow a few minutes for the original owners to write the two strengths that they acknowledge that will help them 'stay on track.'

    7. Problem solve how to use this handout for future motivational support.

Activity handout and facilitator's information submitted by Erika Pond Clements, OT Reg. (Ont.), Dip. Add., Kitchener, Ontario, Canada. Erika, a regular contributor to Life Management Skills publications, is in private practice focusing on mental and behavioral health and addictions issues. Her leisure interests are tai chi and yoga.

My Gift to Me . . .

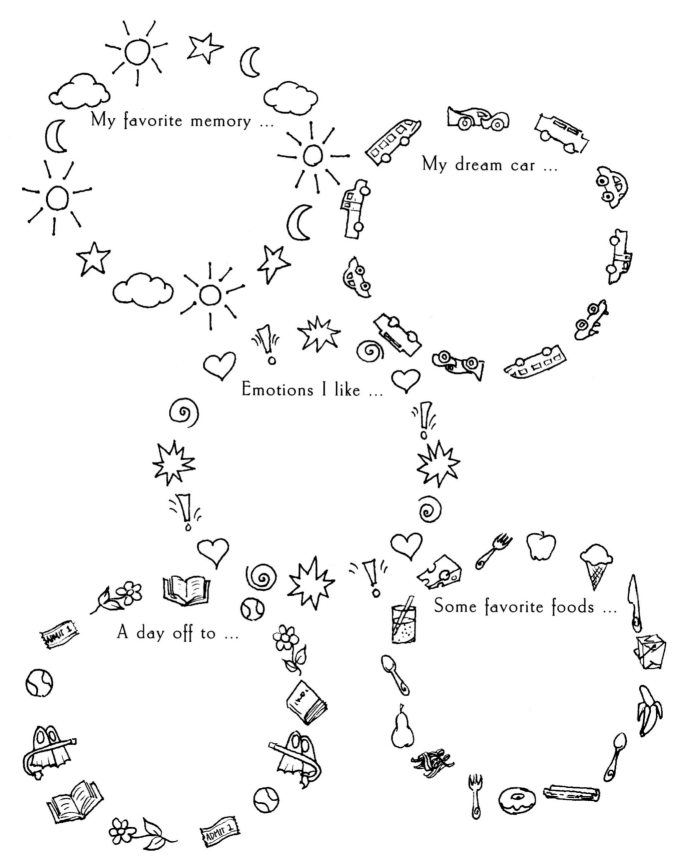

My favorite memory . . .

My dream car . . .

Emotions I like . . .

Some favorite foods . . .

A day off to . . .

My Gift to Me . . .

I. PURPOSE:

To understand the concept of giving to oneself as a means of nurturing and raising self-esteem.

II. GENERAL COMMENTS:

This exercise introduces and/or reinforces the idea of giving to self. Many people need to become more comfortable with the notion that giving to self is okay and appropriate as opposed to 'selfish' or 'conceited.' There are many ways of giving to self – tangibly or otherwise. This might be especially appropriate during stressful times such as holidays, times of trauma and illness.

III. POSSIBLE ACTIVITIES:

A. 1. Introduce session by asking participants to share a great gift they received at some point in their life.

2. Facilitate a discussion on the concept of giving to self, e.g., the value of giving to self, barriers associated with giving to self, and raise the notion of intangible gifts.

3. Distribute handouts and pens. Provide ten to fifteen minutes for participants to complete.

4. Reconvene and allow each participant to share the gifts they wrote about. Ask group members if there were categories not included that could make for good gifts to self (e.g., A visit with…, To listen to…).

5. Have the group discuss some ways to implement the written exercise into some practical ideas.

B. 1. Explain the concept of giving to self. Ask participants to share a personal experience of giving to self. How did it feel at the time? If any participants have never given to self, encourage them to identify what has stopped them from doing so.

2. Distribute handouts and provide ten to fifteen minutes to complete. Play soothing, non-distractible music to add to the self-nurturing atmosphere of the group.

3. Provide time to share findings in sub-groups of two or three. Ask group members to discuss in smaller group if there were categories not included, that could make for good gifts to self (e.g., A visit with…, To listen to…).

4. Reconvene as a larger group to discuss how to take these ideas and implement them to action. It may be necessary to facilitate a discussion on the participants' difficulties or concerns with the concept of giving to self, i.e., being taught at a young age not to be 'selfish' or to always 'put others first'.

5. Discuss idea of finding balance between giving to self and giving to others.

Activity handout and facilitator's information submitted by Nancy Day, BScO.T. Reg (Ont), Markham, Ontario, Canada. Nancy has had 20 of her handouts published in the Life Management Skills series. She provides hospital-based occupational therapy services to clients experiencing mental health problems within a team-oriented program emphasizing group therapies. Nancy's leisure interests are quilting, reading, antiques and hiking.

Positively Positive

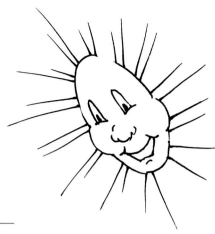

3 things I like about me...

_____
_____
_____

3 things I like about _____ (Fill in person's name – Example: name of Mom, Brother, etc.)

_____
_____
_____

3 things I like about _____ (Fill in person's name)

_____
_____
_____

3 things I like about _____ (Fill in person's name)

_____
_____
_____

3 things I like about _____ (Fill in person's name)

_____
_____
_____

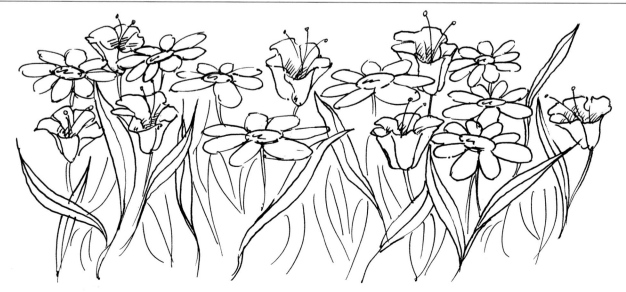

Positively Positive

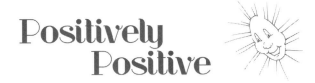

I. PURPOSE:

To promote self-esteem and positive relationships within one's support system.

II. GENERAL COMMENTS:

Sometimes it is difficult to verbally express the positive aspects we like about family members, friends, peers and especially ourselves. It's time that we get these thoughts and feelings out in the open! Hearing and saying positive things about others and ourselves is a valuable skill that has numerous healing benefits.

III. POSSIBLE ACTIVITIES:

A. 1. Instruct group members to sit in a circle.

2. Give group members handouts, pens and clipboards (if not sitting around a table). Ask each person to fill out three things they like about themselves, and also, three things they like about EVERY other person in the group. Distribute as many handouts as necessary.

3. Upon completion of the handout, ask group members to share their feelings during this exercise.

4. Process by asking one or all of the following questions:

   a. "Was it hard to come up with things that you like about yourself?"
   b. "How did it feel to verbalize the positive feelings you have about yourself?"
   c. "How did it feel to say nice, positive things about others?"
   d. "How did it feel to hear nice things about yourself?"

B. 1. Introduce the topic that, for many people, negative thinking is a habit. Seeing the worst in situations, health conditions and people, can seem like a never-ending process in our minds.

2. Discuss the consequences of negative thinking by listing all possibilities on the board.

3. Explain that it is possible to 'look for the good.' Although at times it may feel like 'mining for gold', this skill can be extremely valuable in all aspects of life!

4. Distribute handouts and pencils.

5. Instruct group members to complete handouts by examining personal attributes and admired attributes in others. Give ten minutes for completion.

6. Allow ten minutes for sharing results, feelings associated with the activity, and benefits of 'looking for the good' along with honest expression of positives of self and others in one's life.

Activity handout and facilitator's information submitted by Esterlee A. Molyneux, M.S., SSW, Logan, UT.
Esterlee is a program coordinator. She teaches parenting classes, provides in-home parenting skills, teaches an in-school sexual abuse curriculum, supervises children's anger management and social skills classes. Esterlee's leisure interests are scrapbooking, traveling, making crafts and spending time with family.

_____
_____
_____
_____
_____
_____

Things I am ashamed of:

_____
_____
_____
_____
_____
_____

Things I am proud of:

_____
_____
_____
_____
_____
_____

I would describe myself as:

Things I want to strive for:

_____
_____
_____

Things I can do to feel
better about myself:

_____
_____
_____

The
Story of

_____

The Story of _____

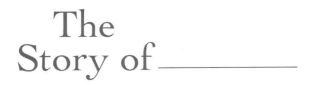

I. PURPOSE:

To increase self-esteem through self-examination.

To develop an appreciation for what is special and unique about each person.

II. GENERAL COMMENTS:

Each of us is the only real expert of our own life and is capable of creating our own solutions. This expressive, creative activity hopes to promote a realistic self-image and offer new insights.

III. POSSIBLE ACTIVITIES:

A. 1. Distribute handouts.

2. Describe the storybook layout and instruct group members to fold paper into fourths.

3. Review the importance of self-awareness and self-esteem.

4. Instruct group members to complete handout, using a variety of pencils, pens, colored markers, etc. They can write words or draw pictures to symbolize their answers.

5. Allow 15-20 minutes for completion.

6. Encourage group members to divide into pairs to share their stories. Create atmosphere of acceptance, support and honest feedback.

7. Reconvene and process similarities and/or differences among the group members.

B. 1. Distribute handouts to group members.

2. Describe the storybook layout and instruct group members to fold paper into fourths.

3. Review the importance of self-awareness and self-esteem. Explain that each of us has a story to tell and that is what makes us unique. Taking time to self-reflect, to see who we are and to actively work on our self-esteem, are life skills that promote growth, strength and resilience.

4. Instruct group members to complete handout, using a variety of pencils, pens, colored markers, etc. They can write words or draw pictures to symbolize their answers. Tell group members that later, others will listen to these stories.

5. Allow 15-20 minutes for completion.

6. Collect the handouts. Read aloud each story and ask group members to try and identify who wrote the story.

7. Process benefits of self-awareness and self-esteem.

Activity handout and facilitator's information submitted by Diana Fain. MOT, OTR/L, Miami, FL.
Diana has worked in both psychiatric and geriatric settings during her pursuit of her master's degree.
Currently she specializes in pediatrics as a school based occupational therapist. Diana's leisure activity is baking!

Who Am I Anyway?

 = giving

 = good observer

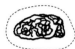 = intelligent

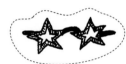 = sense of style

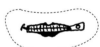 = good at keeping secrets

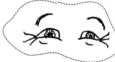 = funny

 = caring

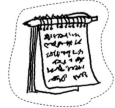 = good writer

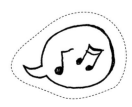 = musically talented

good listener =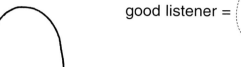

sensitive =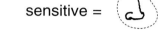

creative =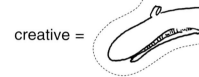

cheery =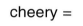

polite =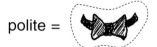

energetic =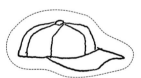

good conversationalist =

good at time management =

athletic =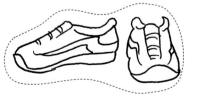

artistically talented =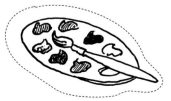

Who Am I Anyway?

I. PURPOSE:
To develop a positive self-image.

II. GENERAL COMMENTS:
This activity encourages recognizing one's self-worth and strengths in a creative and structured format.

III. POSSIBLE ACTIVITIES:
A. 1. Distribute one handout to each individual and make supplies available to all: scissors, markers, crayons, glitter, glue, yarn, and other media choices.
   2. Instruct group members to cut out body and glue on colored paper.
   3. Instruct group members to make a picture of themselves which must include five positive traits. These positive traits may come from the pictures provided, or individuals may draw or depict the traits using creative materials.
   4. Instruct each person to share his/her self-image project and explain the five positive traits chosen.
   5. Provide positive reinforcement by having the group applaud for each person or by having the group give five more positive traits.
   6. Process the activity by asking:
      a. "What did you like/dislike about this activity?"
      b. "Did you find it easy or hard to come up with positive traits about yourself?"
      c. "How did you feel when others told you positive traits about yourself?"

B. 1. Discuss self-image and the lifelong skill of working to maintain a heightened awareness of seeing the positives in ourselves as well as in others. Incorporate idea that what we see in others, we might be able to see in ourselves. As we look for the good in others, we might be able to see the good in ourselves.
   2. Distribute handouts, magazines, glue and scissors.
   3. Instruct group members to cut out body and glue on colored paper.
   4. Ask each person to write his/her name on the colored paper and collect them.
   5. Redistribute them so each person receives another person's handout.
   6. Instruct group members to complete by finding eight positive traits about the individual whose name is on the paper, either from pictures on the handout or words/pictures from magazines.
   7. Ask each individual to stand in front of the group, one-by-one and present his/her 'self-image person.'
   8. Process by asking:
      a. "Why is it important to see the positives in others?"
      b. "How does a positive self-image affect your learning a new skill? At home? In business? With your family? With strangers?"

Activity handout and facilitator's information submitted by Katie Schroeder-Smith, MOT, Frederick, MD.
Katie graduated summa cum laude with her Master of Occupational Therapy degree in January 2002.
She enjoys drawing, painting, crafts, reading, tennis, downhill skiing and kickboxing.

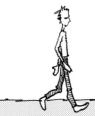

Risking to Learn a New Skill

A Journey of a Thousand Miles Must Begin with a Single Step.

How does the above Chinese proverb relate to skill development? _____

Is it time for you to learn something new? A hobby? A sport? A job skill? What is it? _____

EVERYDAY WE FACE CHALLENGES IN OUR LIVES. Some challenges may be dialing a phone, cooking dinner, or even getting out of bed in the morning. When it comes to learning something new, it may be a difficult challenge. The important thing is to be patient and forgiving with yourself.

Types of challenges you have experienced in your life: _____

How you overcame these challenges: _____

When learning anything new, there may be stress. What are some ways you relieve stress? _____

How can your ability to use humor help you when trying to learn this new skill? _____

DON'T PUT YOURSELF DOWN! PLEASE! Without even realizing it, many of us put ourselves down, call ourselves names, and say things like: "I'm so stupid"; "I can't do anything right"; "Everyone thinks I'm an idiot!" That kind of self-talk really hurts and gets in the way of learning!

When you put yourself down, what do you say? _____

Examples of positive self-talk: _____

POSITIVELY ACCEPTING OURSELVES: An optimistic outlook about learning new things is the key to success! All of us would like to change something about ourselves. If we have a positive outlook on learning new things, we can better accept ourselves. When learning something new, we must first look at our self-acceptance and how it can impact our ability to learn.

Things I would like to change about myself: _____

Things I can't change about myself: _____

How to improve my positive outlook: _____

How can learning new things influence my ability to accept myself? _____

LAUGHTER CAN LIFT OUR SPIRITS AND IMPROVE OUR MENTAL HEALTH. Sometimes it is hard to laugh at ourselves, especially when we make a silly mistake. When we learn something, there is a good chance that we may make a mistake. We need to remember that we can laugh about those things and then move on!

Times I made a mistake: _____

Times when I was able to laugh at myself: _____

Ways I can laugh at myself when I mess up: _____

You're on the way to learning a new skill!

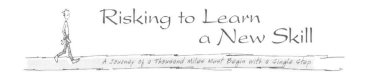

I. PURPOSE:

To examine fears of learning a new skill and to identify the positive and negative ways of dealing with our feelings.

II. GENERAL COMMENTS:

It's easy to give up on new things that we find challenging simply because we are afraid of failing. Thinking about what it takes to learn something new and then dealing with all the thoughts and feelings, is a good way to tackle and succeed!

III. POSSIBLE ACTIVITIES:

A. 1. Distribute handouts and pens.
2. Give group members 10-15 minutes to complete.
3. Discuss.
4. Ask group members to share their challenges and discuss how they overcame them.
5. Question group about stress associated with challenges: "How did you deal with the stress?" "What did you use as stress relievers?" List input from group members on dry-erase board for all to see.
6. Have group members share times when they put themselves down. "What are the triggers?" "What is said?"
7. Discuss examples of self-talk.
8. Ask the group to focus on humor: How can humor affect the way that you approach challenges? Share personal examples, if able, of when you have successfully used humor when confronted with challenges.
9. Encourage members to examine how they deal with challenges of learning a new skill and their thoughts, emotions and feelings surrounding that situation. Process.

B. 1. Distribute handouts and pens.
2. Discuss challenges and obstacles of 'risking to learn a new skill.'
3. Pair group members according to commonalities of challenges or the type of skill to be learned.
4. Ask pairs to come up with their own proverb or saying, to help themselves / others relate to that specific challenge.
5. Take the proverbs or sayings and make a 'Words to Risk By' calendar, to remind each group member that throughout the year, risks can be taken with some encouragement. For example: "Go forth & be risky!"

Activity handout and facilitator's information submitted by Jodi Wilson Overstreet, M.Ed., LPC, NCC, Harrisburg, IL. Jodi manages a three County PSR program for adults with chronic mental illness, providing individual and group therapy, developing educational curriculum and organizing community education. She says "Leisure – what's that? With a son learning to create havoc – I do enjoy cooking, crafts, reading, singing, and remodeling great-grandma's house."

Your Path to Using Skills

- What skill(s) do you want to maintain? _____
- What needs to happen in order to use and remember the skills you have learned?

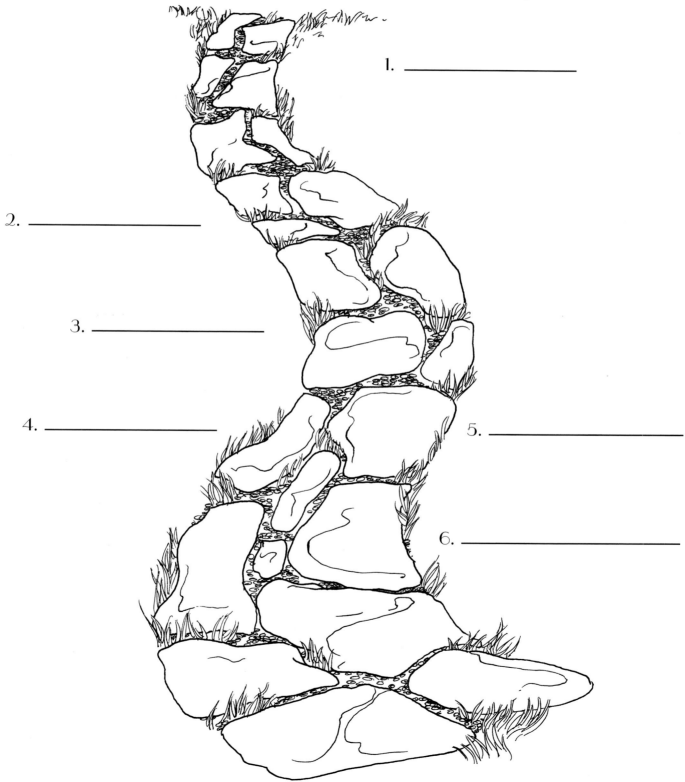

1. _____

2. _____

3. _____

4. _____

5. _____

6. _____

Your Path to Using Skills

I. PURPOSE:

To identify strategies for skills generalization outside of group or treatment.

II. GENERAL COMMENTS:

Many times therapeutic groups are held just once or twice a week. People have identified the difficulty in transferring coping techniques and other skills to outside of the treatment / group environment. It is hoped that by working together and devising strategies for more carryover, skills can be transferred more easily.

III. POSSIBLE ACTIVITIES:

A. 1. List on a dry-erase board the challenges of transferring skills to outside of the treatment setting and discuss.
   2. Develop a second list of the benefits of transferring skills and knowledge to outside of the group. Emphasize the importance of skill generalization.
   3. Distribute handouts and pens.
   4. Instruct group members to write suggestions for using skills outside of the group. Ideas generated might include:
      a. groups held more often each week
      b. more review
      c. homework assignments
      d. folders for information at home as well as group folders for group
      e. having group members' phone numbers for support
      f. more family / group home / residential involvement
      People can write in the spaces after each number and on the 'road', too, if they have more than six suggestions.
   5. Compile a list and discuss with group. What ideas are most helpful to each person?
   6. Distribute a second handout to each group member, so those individuals can fill out a blank sheet with the ideas that are most helpful.
   7. Discuss the steps needed to take to get started and how to support each other in these efforts.
   8. Plan a way to evaluate strategies on a regular basis.

B. 1. List skills that group members want to develop. Ideas may include:
      a. more comfortable with people I meet
      b. better job preparation
      c. keeping a cleaner house
      d. accepting change and moving forward
      e. being involved in a more active leisure life
      f. identifying issues
      g. independence in ADL's
      h. being more assertive
   2. Emphasize to group members that no matter which skill needs to be developed, there are always steps or reminders that can help.
   3. Ask group members to write skill desired on top of page.
   4. Ask each group member to share, if comfortable, which skill is identified.
   5. Then ask group members to volunteer six ways or ideas to remember the things learned to achieve this skill or what needs to happen to develop this skill. Encourage note taking to promote active learning.
   6. Discuss benefits of group problem solving and hearing new ideas for what may seem like an old problem!

Activity handout and facilitator's information submitted by Marty Golub, C.T.R.S., Rochester, NY.
Marty is a dependable friend of Wellness Reproductions & Publishing. He coordinates leisure service delivery in a Continuing Day Treatment Program for individuals with mental illness. He plans, leads and evaluates leisure groups. Marty enjoys bowling, football, crafts, traveling, volunteer activities, exercising, volleyball and visiting family in Chicago.

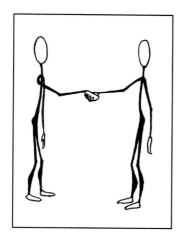

It's a Matter of Manners

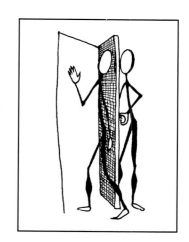

The way we interact with others determines much of our success or failure in our personal and professional lives. Listed below are situations that occur in everyday life. Look at each situation and rate how you would typically act.

Situation	Excellent	Good	Fair	Poor
Eating out				
Meeting new people				
Shopping in a store				
In the doctor's office				
Using the telephone				
Driving in traffic				
At the movies or riding in public transportation				
Talking with your boss or co-workers				
In church, temple, synagogue				
Giving a party				

- Overall, after thinking about and discussing with your peers the situations above, how would you rank your manners?   Excellent ____   Good ____   Fair ____   Poor ____

- How can you go about improving the ways in which you interact with others so that your relationships are much more satisfying? _____

_____

_____

_____

It's a Matter of Manners

I. PURPOSE:

To identify the importance of social skills (manners) in everyday interactions.

II. GENERAL COMMENTS:

It is useful to analyze everyday experiences to determine if one is interacting in a manner that lends itself to success when dealing with others.

III. POSSIBLE ACTIVITIES:

A. 1. Distribute handouts and pens.

   2. Ask group to look at each of the ten situations listed and brainstorm good manners that could be used, e.g., waiting to be seated, thanking the waitress, talking so as not to disturb others eating near you, leaving a tip to reward good service. Write suggestions on a blackboard.

   3. Discuss the effect our manners have on those with whom we interact daily.

   4. Give group members five minutes to complete handouts rating personal manners.

   5. Share ideas in bottom section for improving interaction skills.

B. 1. Cut the ten situations listed on the handout into strips. Place in a basket.

   2. Have each group member choose one strip and list two good manners that could be used in that setting, e.g., speak politely with the clerk, wait your turn.

   3. Ask two group members to role-play manners, e.g., one can be the doctor, one the patient.

   4. Process by discussing how the manners used in each situation may affect our future relationship with those with whom we interact and how we may feel about ourselves as a result of our skills in dealing with others.

Activity handout and facilitator's information submitted by Roberta J. Ott, COTA, M.Ed., Allentown, PA.
Roberta is a Therapeutic Activity Services Worker, providing programs to adult psychiatric patients, e.g., arts, crafts, music, coping skills and life skill development as well as community trips to prepare for discharge. Her leisure interests are tole painting and reading.

Socially Accepted Behaviors... or not!

	INAPPROPRIATE	APPROPRIATE	CONSEQUENCES OR RESULTS
APPEARANCE			
Clothing			
1. Weather Appropriate			
2. Fit			
3. Matched or Coordinated			
4. Cleanliness			
5. Condition			
6. Occasion Appropriate Outfit			
Hygiene			
1. Hair Care			
2. Oral Care			
3. Deodorant			
4. Cologne			
5. Skin Care (make up)			
SOCIAL SKILLS			
1. Greetings			
2. Introduction			
3. Disclosures			
4. Manners			
5. Voice Tone			
6. Criticism			
7. Fault Finding			
8. Obscene Language			
9. Compliments			
10. Listening			
11. Eye Contact			
12. Humor			
13. Nonverbal			
14. Interruption			
PHYSICAL CONTACT			
1. Personal Space			
2. Hug			
3. Touching			
4. Pats			
5. Finger Pointing			
6. Fisting			

Socially Accepted Behaviors...
or not!

I.   PURPOSE:
To increase awareness of the difference between acceptable and nonacceptable behaviors.

II. GENERAL COMMENTS:
For those with psychosocial challenges, social skills and recognizing socially accepted behaviors vs. unacceptable behaviors could be a real challenge. The lack of these skills often results in poor social relations, and at times can lead to isolation and loneliness.

III. POSSIBLE ACTIVITIES:

A. 1. Introduce concept of importance of recognizing socially accepted behaviors. Discuss possible reasons why people might do poorly in this area. (Too sick to notice these details, not taught these skills as children, poor concentration, etc.)
2. Distribute handouts and pens.
3. Read the following letter and situations aloud. Ask group members to place letter in correct box. Use a. as an example to do together.
    a. 'Sitting next to someone whose hair is greasy' would result in the letter A marked in the inappropriate column in the row marked 'Hair Care.'
    b. Someone wearing clothes too tight.
    c. A boss reacting to someone coming to a job interview for a desk job in an evening gown.
    d. Going to a lunch with a friend whose blouse is all stained.
    e. A friend wearing a heavy jacket in summer.
    f. Washing face daily.
    g. Sitting in a restaurant in back of someone whose perfume is too strong.
    h. Going to a party and the host introduces you to the other guests.
    i. Sitting next to a person you just met, and that person telling you their problems.
    j. Someone talking too loud in the movies.
    k. Your friend complimenting you on how you look.
    l. Your next door neighbor screaming and cursing you out, because you took her newspaper by mistake.
    m. Someone you barely know greets you with a bear hug.
    n. Someone putting his or her fist up to your face because of a comment you made.
    o. Someone you barely know making sexually explicit advances towards you.
    p. Your sister doesn't let you get a word in during a discussion.
4. Discuss all consequences and results.
5. Ask group members to circle any areas they feel could use improvement. Allow sharing if this level of disclosure is comfortable and/or desired.
6. Discuss ways of improving these areas.

B. 1. Develop creative way to demonstrate both acceptable and unacceptable social behaviors through skits (possibly generated by clients or staff) or clips from TV shows or movies. Use handout as a guide for behaviors to be discussed.
2. Distribute handouts and pens.
3. Discuss each item separately and thoroughly so all group members understand each behavior.
4. Explain that at times, it's easier to see socially acceptable or unacceptable behaviors in others rather than in ourselves.
5. Show the skits or clips, asking group members to indicate observations on handout.
6. Review as a group and discuss consequences or results of noted behaviors.
7. Allow time for role-plays of the more difficult skills.
8. Facilitate problem solving or goal setting, as indicated by personal disclosures.

Activity handout and facilitator's information submitted by Joan Rascati, A.S. Human Services, East Haven, CT.
Joan has been employed at a mental health agency for many years, teaching and developing social, community and independent living skills programs - and also runs a women's health group. In Joan's leisure time she develops new ways to present material to different groups with different levels of functioning and is also interested in the arts.

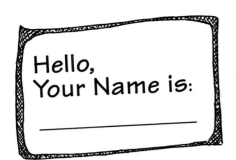

Hello,
Your Name is:
_____

Using and Remembering Names

Using peoples' names in conversation is an effective social and communication skill that can strengthen relationships. It shows friendliness and adds to the warmth of an interaction. What is another reason to use a name in conversation?

_____

_____

_____

How to Remember Names

Many people struggle with remembering names. Here are some strategies:

Just admit you have forgotten. Your honesty will likely be appreciated by the other person who will then provide you with his/her name.

"I'm sorry, I've forgotten your name..."

Other suggestions:

_____
_____
_____
_____

Remind the other person of your name first. This often triggers them to offer their name as well.

"We met last week, I'm Nancy..."

Other suggestions:

_____
_____
_____
_____
_____

Use humor!
"I guess I'm having one of those memory moments – I can't seem to remember your name ..."

Other suggestions:

_____
_____
_____
_____

How to Use Names

Use names in a natural way - either at the beginning, middle or end of the sentence.
Here are some examples:

"Hi Sue, how was your weekend?"
"Thanks for the help, Mike."
"Guess what, Mason, I passed the test!"
"That's a good point, Kim."

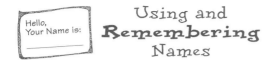

I. PURPOSE:

To learn and practice the social skills of using and remembering names in conversation.

II. GENERAL COMMENTS:

Individuals with psychosocial challenges in their lives often have deficits in social functioning. This, coupled with symptoms such as poor concentration and attention span, can hamper a person's ability to recall names. Using and remembering names is a communication skill important in improving quality of life. The skill of using names in conversation can be learned fairly easily and most people are pleased to quickly experience positive results in social interactions.

III. POSSIBLE ACTIVITIES:

A. 1. Introduce yourself by name and then allow all group members to introduce themselves by name.

2. Ask if anyone can remember all the group members' names and then, do so. Discuss the importance of this skill.

3. Distribute handouts and pencils.

4. Review information presented, along with group members' input and ideas.

5. Offer the following potential role-plays for participants (or use role-plays from the group) to practice using and remembering names:

   a. party introduction with three or four people
   b. meeting someone at AA event
   c. sitting next to a fellow client at an outpatient setting
   d. meeting a specialist on your health care team

6. Emphasize that both skills, using AND remembering names, are useful in a variety of settings.

7. Process by asking group members to turn over handouts, trying to recall what was covered in today's session.

B. 1. Explain that today's session will be divided into two skills: using and remembering names.

2. Discuss relevance of these skills in personal, social and business situations. Reflect on what happens when these skills are NOT used.

3. Distribute handouts and pencils.

4. Review and elicit input from group members about skills or tricks they use to remember names effectively.

5. Divide group into pairs. Have each pair develop three 2-line skits using skills covered. For example: "Sue, what's new with you?" "Not much has happened, Paul, since I saw you last week."

6. Instruct each pair to present their three brief skits.

7. Review that these skills, like all others, require practice.

8. Ask each pair to process one tip learned from this experience and an idea they can use in the future.

Activity handout and facilitator's information submitted by Nancy Day, BScO.T. Reg (Ont), Markham, Ontario, Canada. Nancy has had 20 of her handouts published in the Life Management Skills series. She provides hospital-based occupational therapy services to clients experiencing mental health problems within a team-oriented program emphasizing group therapies. Nancy's leisure interests are quilting, reading, antiques and hiking.

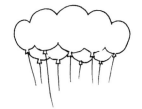

Adding Our Spirit to the Balance:
Developing a
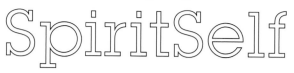

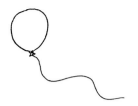

Life is full of emotions, feelings and experiences.
Our emotions and feelings are neutral – they are expressions of who we are as humans. They are our spirit's way of alerting us to how our inner world is interacting with the outer world. It is important to live our life with balance. Investing in our SPIRITUALITY can help us with achieving this balance.

> **To Live Life to the Fullest...**
> **We Need not Fear Our Spirituality but Rather Incorporate it into Who We Are.**
> **And What We Do!**

When you think of the words Spirit, Spiritual, and Spirituality, what images, words, or experiences come to mind?

Picture Your Spiritual Self like a Balloon

Some experiences are negative and act on our spirit like deflating the balloon - they decrease energy. Others are more positive, life giving and supportive and are like inflating the balloon. They strengthen and fill us with energy and support. By the deflated balloons, write what drains your spirit of life and light. By the inflated balloons, write what helps your spirit feel full of life and supported.

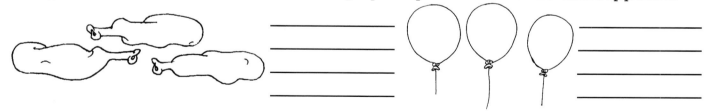

List Tools to Develop Your SpiritSelf

Sacred Place	Special Ritual / Music	Reading Inspirational	Caring Community	Special Friend / Mentor

Create Nurturing Goals

Inner Self	Outer Self	Activities	Places	Other

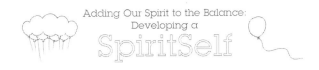

Adding Our Spirit to the Balance: Developing a SpiritSelf

I.   PURPOSE:

To explore and list spiritual activities and determine which ones provide energy and strength and which ones deplete us.

To develop a spiritual self to enhance recovery efforts.

II.   GENERAL COMMENTS:

Differing spiritual practices, situations and experiences produce differing feelings and emotions.
To live life to the fullest, we need to incorporate our spirituality into who we are and what we do.
Developing space for our spirit can be life affirming for those who question or have lost hope.

III.   POSSIBLE ACTIVITIES:

A. 1.   Introduce concept of what is a SpiritSelf – a person who has developed a place in their lives for spirituality to reside and for the spirit to gain strength to be present through life's joys and challenges.

2.   Distribute handouts, regular black and colored pencils. Read introductory paragraphs together.

3.   Instruct group members to complete image box individually.

4.   Review balloon concept by bringing two balloons into the session, one deflated, one inflated. List on board words typically associated with the deflated balloon: tired, sad, flimsy, shriveled, worn, weathered, exhausted, etc. Then, words associated with the inflated balloon: ready-to-go, full of energy, full, happy, perky, peppy, etc. Ask group members if they can relate to the metaphor of our SpiritSelf being like a balloon.

5.   Instruct group members to complete bottom section individually.

6.   Share responses if group members are comfortable.

7.   Process by asking what was gained in this session.

B. 1.   Ask the group members how they view spirituality in respect to faith, healing and wellness.

2.   List the pros and cons of engaging in spiritually enriching activities and spiritually depleting activities.

3.   Distribute handouts, colored pencils and pens.

4.   Give group ten minutes to complete the entire handout except the bottom sections, TOOLS TO DEVELOP OUR SPIRITSELF and NURTURING GOALS.

5.   Divide group into pairs. Allow ten minutes for each person to support the other in completing this bottom section.

6.   Reconvene and ask each individual to report on an interesting tool his/her partner listed to develop the SpiritSelf or on an inspiring goal.

7.   Close the group by reading an inspiring favorite quote, poem or saying that directly relates to the SpiritSelf.

Activity handout and facilitator's information submitted by Reverend Donald Shields, BRE, MTS, CAPPE Certified Specialist in Spiritual and Religious Care; D. Min Candidate, Markham, Ontario, Canada. As the coordinator of spiritual and religious care, Donald facilitates care of patients, volunteers and staff at a 200-bed acute care hospital. He works as part of the mental health team in developing and co-facilitating an inpatient humor group and an outpatient monthly spirituality workshop wherein spirituality is profiled as an ingredient in recovery. He is married with two daughters attending university and enjoys reading, music, movies, caring for and playing with his 3 dogs and 2 cats.

The Desert as a Spiritual Theme

Today we will look at spiritual dryness ... those times when we feel dry, alone, deserted and isolated. The image of the desert is sometimes used by spiritual traditions to describe this experience.

> **What words and images come to mind as you think about a place like the desert?**

At times like this it may be difficult to feel connected to other people or something larger than ourselves. Many others have felt this way also. "Spiritual drought" is a common experience that others too have felt.

Having things to sustain you in the 'desert' are worth exploring, as they are fundamental in surviving and healing.

> **What may sustain you in the spiritual desert?**

> **What lessons might be learned from a journey through the desert?**

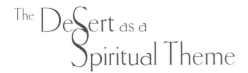

I. PURPOSE:

To increase the concept of spiritual dryness and develop ideas as to what sustains us there.

II. GENERAL COMMENTS:

Mental and physical illness may lead to times of spiritual dryness, commonly called the *spiritual desert*. This activity strives to normalize this experience and develop coping plans in the journey through the *spiritual desert*.

III. POSSIBLE ACTIVITIES:

A. 1. Bring a small amount of sand and encourage members to handle the sand in their hands. Ask for comments on what insights the texture and feel of the sand brings to mind.

2. Present meaningful poems or spiritual writings that describe the experiences of others that have felt dry in the spiritual journey – being sensitive to the participants' backgrounds, cultural and spiritual diversity.

3. Distribute handouts, pens and colored pencils to group members. Read handouts, discuss as needed and encourage participation.

4. Share responses in a supportive atmosphere.

B. 1. Distribute handouts, pens and colored pencils.

2. Read together entire handout as a group and discuss.

3. Share other meaningful poetry or use Eric Clapton's lyrics, <u>You Were There</u> and <u>Tears in Heaven</u>.

4. Instruct group members to complete handouts.

5. Ask group members to draw a spiritual oasis on the reverse side of the handout, and to visually draw images of what might be there to sustain them. Assure group members that art work is not the goal of the session, but the process involved that is.

6. Ask group members to share the drawings and explain.

7. Process by asking group members what was gained from this session and what will they walk away with that will help them?

Activity handout and facilitator's information submitted by Reverend Donald Shields, BRE, MTS, CAPPE Certified Specialist in Spiritual and Religious Care; D. Min Candidate, Markham, Ontario, Canada. As the coordinator of spiritual and religious care, Donald facilitates care of patients, volunteers and staff at a 200-bed acute care hospital. He works as part of the mental health team in developing and co-facilitating an inpatient humor group and an outpatient monthly spirituality workshop wherein spirituality is profiled as an ingredient in recovery. He is married with two daughters attending university and enjoys reading, music, movies, caring for and playing with his 3 dogs and 2 cats.

Stumbling towards the light:

The Spiritual Journey

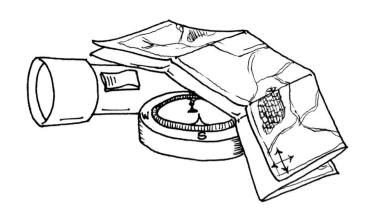

What Is a Spiritual Journey?

The spiritual journey or 'journey of the spirit' is a common quest that we find ourselves on. It is a quest for understanding and meaning. It is a quest to make sense of joy and suffering and all that takes place between the two.

> *Reflection:* Some people refer to the beginnings of the spiritual journey as originating from a crisis of faith. What crisis could initiate a spiritual journey in our lives?

Packing for the Journey:

As in any other journey, the journey of the spirit is not without its needs for supplies and luggage. The journey can be disorientating and confusing so there may be a need for a compass and a map. Times of isolation and sadness can be cold and windy. Items to provide warmth and shelter come in handy. Supplies for celebrations of unique discoveries about others and ourselves are also important!

> *Reflection:* Playing with the metaphor of 'packing for the journey' – what might a compass for the spiritual journey look like? What things could nurture us and provide warmth on the spiritual journey?

The Journey Not the Destination

The spiritual journey is unique because the journey is much more important than the destination. It is through the journey that we arrive at a destination, yet if we focus too much on the destination, we can fail to observe the scenery of the journey. We do not want to lose sight of the lessons along the journey's path.

> *Reflection:* What are some lessons that we may learn on our spiritual journey?

The Spiritual Journey

I. PURPOSE:

To facilitate defining a personal 'spiritual journey.'

II. GENERAL COMMENTS:

Life's difficulties, such as health problems and losses, can precipitate a 'crisis of faith' that becomes the point of demarcation for the beginning of a spiritual journey for answers to life's great questions: "Who am I?" "What does this mean?" "Is there more or is this all there is?" This activity will facilitate discussion of the spiritual journey.

CAUTION: Be sure not to engage clients who may be experiencing religious delusions and whose condition could be compromised by the nature of this activity.

III. POSSIBLE ACTIVITIES:

A. 1. Distribute handouts, markers and pens.
2. Introduce topic of 'spiritual journeys' using GENERAL COMMENTS as a guideline.
3. Review handouts with group members, giving ample time to complete reflections boxes.
4. Find fitting poetry or lyrics that would add to the understanding of the topic. One idea is *A Song for the Journey (Observations of a Fellow Traveler) I Want to Live,* by John Denver.
5. Discuss implications of being with others that are also on a spiritual journey and the importance of community for support and healing.

B. 1. Distribute handouts, markers and pens.
2. Review handouts with group members by first reading through the handout and then giving ten minutes to illustrate reflections boxes using words or drawing images.
3. Discuss and look at completed handouts.
4. Provide blank paper for collages along with magazine pictures of camping, backpacking or any other travel images.
5. Instruct group members to design a collage using cut out pictures and ask them to label what is needed for the spiritual journey.
6. Provide a resource list of websites and community resources to enable people to pursue the spiritual journey.
7. Focus on the unique nature of each person's spiritual journey.

Activity handout and facilitator's information submitted by Reverend Donald Shields, BRE, MTS, CAPPE Certified Specialist in Spiritual and Religious Care; D. Min Candidate, Markham, Ontario, Canada. As the coordinator of spiritual and religious care, Donald facilitates care of patients, volunteers and staff at a 200-bed acute care hospital. He works as part of the mental health team in developing and co-facilitating an inpatient humor group and an outpatient monthly spirituality workshop wherein spirituality is profiled as an ingredient in recovery. He is married with two daughters attending university and enjoys reading, music, movies, caring for and playing with his 3 dogs and 2 cats.

A BALANCED Lifestyle

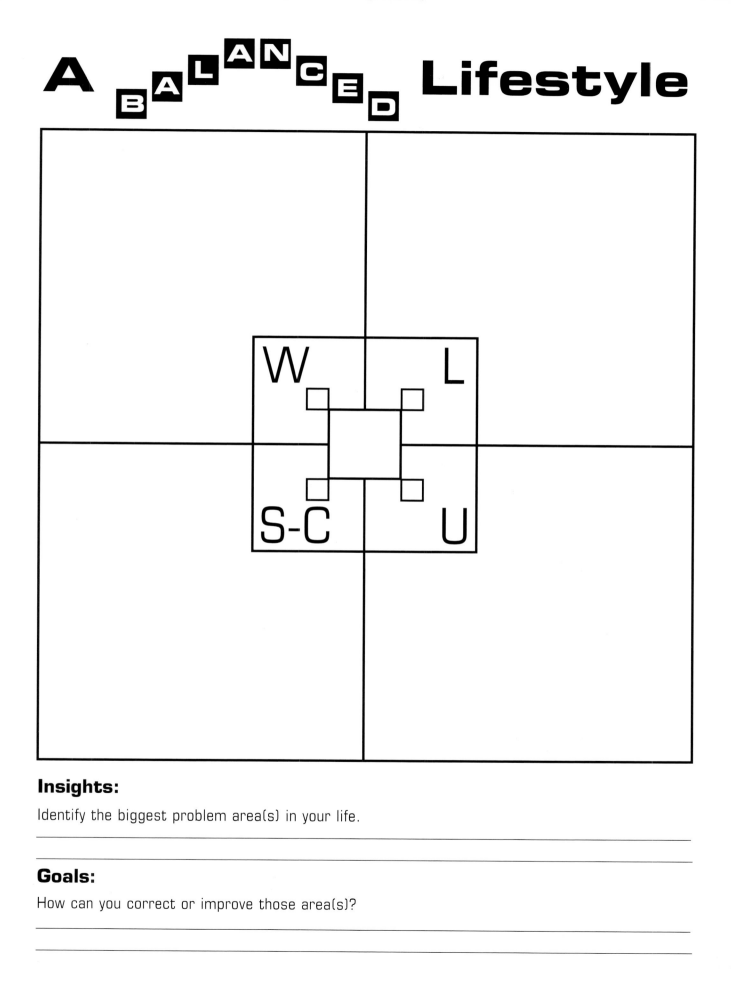

Insights:

Identify the biggest problem area(s) in your life.

_____

_____

Goals:

How can you correct or improve those area(s)?

_____

_____

A 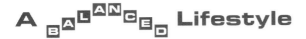 Lifestyle

I. PURPOSE:

To identify how an individual's time is spent in the four areas of one's life (work, leisure, self-care and the unhealthy).

To improve time management by identifying leisure possibilities and/or changes needed for a healthier lifestyle.

II. GENERAL COMMENTS:

When areas of one's life become unbalanced, the possibilities of relapse, hospitalization, rehabilitation, incarceration and/or death are very real outcomes. A balanced lifestyle between work, leisure and self-care improves an individual's ability to cope with stress, allowing one to become productive, positive, healthier and happier in all aspects of one's life: spiritually, mentally, emotionally and physically.

III. POSSIBLE ACTIVITIES:

A. 1. Discuss time management in relation to life balance and imbalance.

   2. Distribute handouts and pens to group members.

   3. Instruct members to write in each specific block, ONLY those activities they were actually doing prior to hospitalization, using the following guidelines: Break down each category and list on the board: work, leisure, self-care and unhealthy.

     a. WORK: activities you have to do – may/may not enjoy them
       examples: job, housework, errands, shopping, budgeting, cooking, paying bills

     b. LEISURE: activities you do that are fun, relaxing and/or enriching that are healthy for you
       examples: sports, hobbies, arts/crafts, TV, music, pets, visiting with friends

     c. SELF-CARE: activities that are vital to your health and well-being
       examples: sleep, medication, relaxation, eating, spirituality, support groups, goals

     d. UNHEALTHY: activities and/or behaviors you do that are unhealthy
       examples: drugs, alcohol, self-pity, negative relations, excessive TV

   4. Inform members, by doing an unhealthy behavior while engaged in a healthy activity, the negative behavior cancels out the positive behavior. Have the group members adjust their blocks accordingly.

   5. Instruct group members to calculate how many hours they spend in each category, on an average weekday, prior to treatment. This total goes in the inside corner boxes (not the center box).

   6. Instruct group members to add the four numbers and place the sum in the center box.

   7. Emphasize to group members that there are only 24 hours in a day. If an individual has less than 24 for the sum, the missing hours will most likely fall into the unhealthy category. If an individual has more than 24 for the sum, there was an exaggeration or over-estimation made in one of the categories.

   8. Instruct group members to complete the bottom of the page.

   9. Encourage sharing of totals and changes that need to be made.

  10. Process the discussed information, benefits of the activity and encourage goal attainment.

B. 1. Distribute two handouts to each group member.

   2. Follow POSSIBLE ACTIVITY A. 1. through 6.

   3. Have members share findings and the totals in their blocks.

   4. Instruct participants to complete the second handout with the specific changes they would like to make for a healthier lifestyle, omitting the bottom section.

   5. Have members share feelings on both handouts, along with any insights or realizations. Problem solve ways to make these changes happen.

   6. Process the benefits of this activity.

Activity handout and facilitator's information submitted by Kimberly White, CTRS, Hale Center, TX.
Kimberly developed a therapeutic recreation program seven years ago at a facility that specializes in mental health and chemical dependency issues. She provides groups on leisure education, relaxation therapy, time management and life management skills. Kimberly genuinely cares about her patients and focuses on teaching them how to reduce stressors and better manage their lives.

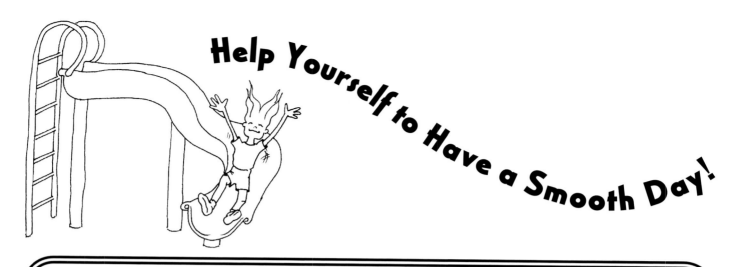

Help Yourself to Have a Smooth Day!

A day goes much more smoothly, with considerably less stress, if we utilize our time wisely. Following each statement below, place a "T" if the statement is true (you do this on a regular basis). Place an "F" if the statement is false (you do NOT do this on a regular basis). After discussing these nine suggestions, think of three more of your own to add to this list of timesaving strategies.

1. To save time getting ready in the morning, I lay out clothing the night before. _____

2. I pack my lunch the night before. _____

3. I set my alarm to go off 15 minutes early. _____

4. When not using them, I keep my keys in the same place at all times. _____

5. I arrive at my appointment / job a few minutes early. _____

6. On my way home, I run errands so I don't have to make a special trip out later in the day. _____

7. When cleaning my apartment / home, I do one room a day. _____

8. I use a calendar to keep track of important events. _____

9. I make up a "To Do" list each weekend for the following week. _____

10. _____ _____

11. _____ _____

12. _____ _____

HOPE YOU HAVE A SMOOTH ONE!

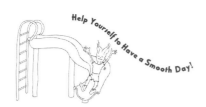
Help Yourself to Have a Smooth Day!

I. **PURPOSE:**

To identify strategies to handle time wisely.

II. **GENERAL COMMENTS:**

It is useful to analyze how we use our time during any given day. There are techniques we can utilize which will make our day go smoothly, thus reducing some of life's stress and helping us to have a more balanced life.

III. **POSSIBLE ACTIVITIES:**

A. 1. Ask group to brainstorm ways in which they save time. Write these on a flipchart, e.g. use paper plates, wash clothes only in large loads, cook in large quantities and then freeze portions.

2. Distribute handouts and pens.

3. Give group several minutes to read and complete the handout.

4. Share results and any techniques the group members added at #10, 11 and 12.

5. Discuss importance of handling time wisely.

B. 1. Distribute handouts and pens.

2. Ask group members to complete handouts.

3. Divide into subgroups of two or three group members.

4. Ask each subgroup to brainstorm ways time can be saved at home, on the job or on weekends. Foster healthy competition by offering a small treat to the subgroup that gets the most ideas or perhaps original ideas.

5. Reconvene as a large group and share findings.

6. Process the importance of using time wisely in order to maintain a balanced life.

Activity handout and facilitator's information submitted by Roberta J. Ott, COTA, M.Ed., Allentown, PA.
Roberta is a Therapeutic Activity Services Worker, providing programs to adult psychiatric patients, e.g., arts, crafts, music, coping skills and life skill development as well as community trips to prepare for discharge.
Her leisure interests are tole painting and reading.

TIME ON MY HANDS

EACH ACTIVITY THAT WE DO TAKES TIME IN OUR DAY.

Routine activities such as commuting, eating, work, sleep and school become part of our regular schedule automatically. Other activities such as exercise, shopping and household chores need to be scheduled around our routine activities. And then we fit other activities such as recreation and socializing into our free time! Take time to consider how much time you spend in different activities. Take time to consider what you would do if you had a set amount of time for certain activities.

What do you do (or COULD you do) with your time?

Activities of Daily Living	Work & Productivity	Rest	Leisure

TIME ON MY HANDS

I. PURPOSE:

To increase awareness of what one may do with different amounts of time.

II. GENERAL COMMENTS:

Time management is a difficult life skill for most people; those who are employed, those who are unemployed, parents, retirees, even college students, all struggle with 'getting it all in.' Living a balanced lifestyle has tremendous health benefits as well as contributing to a high degree of life satisfaction.

III. POSSIBLE ACTIVITIES:

A. 1. Introduce topic of time management and the importance of a balance of activities.

2. Distribute handouts and pens.

3. Bring a deck of regular playing cards for the activity and remove all picture cards (jacks, queens and kings).

4. Identify which types of cards correspond with which activity categories and write on board.
For example: diamonds = work and productivity   hearts = rest
                    spade = ADL (activities of daily living)   clubs = leisure

5. Pass the deck of cards around for each person to select the top card.

6. Have each person reveal his or her card, identifying the category and number of hours for the activity. Then, each person needs to identify what specific activity s/he would do during that amount of time. NOTE: Different group members may list the same activity under different headings (e.g., walking could be considered an ADL as exercise or LEISURE). Each member should decide how to categorize the activities and what amount of time is spent with each. Particularly with the longer time periods (e.g., 5+ hours), most group members will not be able to identify activities that they do for that long. They should be encouraged to use creativity and to group similar types of activities to fill the time (e.g., 5 hours of ADL could include a MORNING FOR ME: taking a long bath, pampering myself, doing my nails). More creative answers may need to be reviewed for how realistic the person's resources are. To eliminate this problem, the group leader may remove cards with higher numbers.

7. Instruct each person to write the activities and number of hours s/he selected in the appropriate category. List the activities on a writing board for all to see.

8. Continue until deck is used up or time allows.

9. Process by asking group members what was learned or if any changes can be considered, after looking at their daily activities in a new way.

B. 1. Discuss how we select activities that we do, what or who influences the decisions we make, and how we organize our time.

2. Distribute handouts and pens. Ask each person to complete the actual schedule by listing the activities they currently do and writing the hours devoted to each. For example, in the ADL category, one person may write 1 hour shower and get dressed, 8 hours of sleep, 1/2 hour of exercise.

3. Share insights.

4. Bring a deck of regular playing cards for the activity and remove all picture cards (jacks, queens and kings). Separate the cards by suit.

5. Identify which types of cards correspond with which activity categories and write on board.
For example: diamonds = work and productivity   hearts = rest
                    spade = ADL (activities of daily living)   clubs = leisure

6. Distribute pencils or different color pens. Ask each group member to select one card from each suit. (See NOTE in A. 6. above)

7. Using the number of hours for each category, ask the group members to write the activities that they COULD do for that amount of time for each category.

8. Process by asking group members if this activity was helpful at looking at schedules in a new way.

Activity handout and facilitator's information submitted by K. Oscar Larson, OTL, MA, BCG, Alexandria, VA.
Oscar coordinates therapeutic activities in an acute psychiatric hospital with a partial hospital program. His leisure interests are gardening, theatre, hiking, reading and art – and has his handouts published in Life Management Skills IV, V, VI and now VII.

Time to Delegate?

10 QUESTIONS THAT WILL REVEAL YOUR THOUGHTS ABOUT DELEGATING.

Briefly describe a task you are considering delegating:

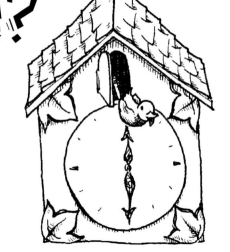

_____

_____

Ask yourself the following questions to determine whether this task could be delegated.
Record your responses in the space provided.

1 Does this task really need to be done?   YES ⬭   NO ⬭
Why? _____

2 Can someone else do it?   YES ⬭   NO ⬭
Who? _____

3 Do I want to do it?   YES ⬭   NO ⬭
Why? / Why not? _____

4 Is it important for me to do it?   YES ⬭   NO ⬭
Why? / Why not? _____

5 Is this something I have to do?   YES ⬭   NO ⬭
If yes, then list reasons why: _____

6 What is the worst thing that can happen if it doesn't get done? _____

7 Who will mind if this doesn't get done? _____

8 If I choose to do it, who can help? _____

9 Can I pay someone else to do it?   YES ⬭   NO ⬭

10 What would I gain if I hire or ask someone else to do it? _____

_____

Time to Delegate?

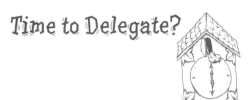

I. PURPOSE:

To increase time management skills by:
- learning to delegate tasks when appropriate
- learning a self-questioning method to reduce the anxiety of incomplete tasks at home or at work

II. GENERAL COMMENTS:

It is easy to say we can delegate tasks to family members, co-workers or committee members, but it's much harder to actually do. Obstacles to effective delegating may include irrational beliefs, fears, and lack of knowledge on how to delegate. Awareness of the benefits, as well as the pitfalls to delegating a specific task may give us the information we need to make the important decision of whether or not to delegate.

III. POSSIBLE ACTIVITIES:

A. 1. Brainstorm and list tasks that seem to cause feelings of worry or anxiety because they are not getting done. Make two separate lists: one for work tasks (e.g. filing, projects, memos) and one for home or personal tasks (e.g., doing laundry, tax preparation, paying the bills, grocery shopping, cleaning garage).
2. Explain delegating as a time management tool.
3. Distribute handouts and pens.
4. Ask participants to choose a task from either list and write a brief description of the task at the top of the handout, e.g., grocery shopping.
5. Using that description, have participants read the questions and record their responses on the handout.
6. Share discoveries and / or decisions of whether or not to delegate in small groups.
7. Reconvene as a larger group and process obstacles and benefits of delegating.

B. 1. Discuss time management as a tool for managing stress. Give real-life examples, show comics or clips from movies to dramatize the point.
2. Explain the use of appropriate delegation of tasks as one time management strategy.
3. Brainstorm with group reasons we tend not to delegate tasks. Record the reasons on the board or flipchart, e.g., fear, maintain control, lack of time, too much work.
4. Distribute handouts and pens.
5. Choose one task (at work or at home) that is not getting done, yet is important. Walk through the problem-solving questions asking group members to write responses to each question on the handout.
6. Share discoveries and decisions of whether to delegate this task or not.
7. Ask group members to flip over the handout so they can't see the front. Explain that one value to a self-questioning method is that we can use it all the time, by ourselves, but we need to try and remember the questions. Elicit questions remembered from the front of the handout and write on a flipchart.

Activity handout and facilitator's information submitted by Nina Beth Sellner, M. Ed., Owatonna, MN.
Nina is a Health Promotion Associate and teaches stress management classes and provides wellness education for employees through handouts, awareness bulletins and presentations. She sets up exercise programs for employees, monitoring their progress. Nina enjoys reading, biking, cross-country skiing and collecting snowmen and celebrity autographs. She is active with her local church in children's ministries and the local toastmaster's club.

Personal
Recovery Packet

I recognize that recovery takes work.
It takes strength, resources and support.
It takes self-acceptance and insight.
It takes knowledge.
The recovery process takes time, energy and patience.
Recovery is a commitment I make to myself.

_____'s

Personal Recovery Packet

About The *Personal Recovery Packet*

This reproducible, supplemental section, entitled *The Personal Recovery Packet*, is designed to be used either in its entirety or as individual handouts.

Its purpose is to provide each client an opportunity to develop a notebook or folder of a personalized and individualized nature to support concepts basic to recovery. This packet promotes opportunities for learning, self-acceptance and for the development of insight.

As health care professionals present information, it is important to ask ourselves several key questions: how much of the information we present is retained? Understood? Relevant? Accepted? Meaningful? The format of this packet empowers the client to rephrase, paraphrase and write in a language that s / he uses. In this way, the packet is the client's (and not the health care professional's). We, as health care professionals, will have the opportunity to receive input from the clients – we will be able to observe first-hand what the clients are writing and hear their questions and concerns. This will help to identify what we need to adapt so we can maximize client benefit.

Folders or notebooks are a great way to organize this packet and can be given to the client at the beginning of a program. Other information you might want to include in the folder or notebook may include medication sheets, other Life Management Skills activity handouts, brochures about the facility or program, book lists, etc.

A multi-disciplinary team can utilize this packet. Professionals can divide up the topics and work collaboratively to ensure addressing different aspects of recovery:

> About My Diagnosis
> About My Symptoms
> About My Medications
> About My Coping Strategies
> About My Supports
> About My Strengths
> About My Area(s) That Need Improvement
> About My Resources

Multiple sheets may be issued when indicated, e.g., someone may have two diagnoses and would need two handouts titled "About My Diagnosis." This packet can be used for education and to meet patient education requirements at your facility. This tool may be assistive in developing client-centered goals.

The ***Ideas for How-to-Use*** on the back of the handouts are for you, the facilitator, and meant to be used 'as is' or to spark and generate ideas for you to develop a meaningful activity for your clients.

IDEAS FOR HOW TO USE THE COVER SHEET:

1. Review intent of packet.
2. Encourage creative expression (highlighters, colored pencils, glitter).
3. Allow different clients to read cover page affirmations prior to each session.

About My Diagnosis

A diagnosis is a medical term that characterizes an illness / disorder by signs and symptoms. It is not meant to be a label that identifies a type of person. You <u>have</u> a diagnosis, but <u>you</u> are <u>not</u> your diagnosis.

The name of my diagnosis is: _____.

That means that: _____
_____
_____.

I have had this diagnosis since: (approximate date) _____.

Circle correct response:
I am the only one in my family with this diagnosis. OR
There are other people in my family with this diagnosis.

My illness / disorder is usually treated by: (List all treatments)
_____
_____
_____
_____
_____
_____

Other information:
_____
_____
_____
_____
_____

About My Diagnosis

IDEAS FOR HOW-TO-USE

1. Bring medical book with diagnosis information, fact sheets off the Internet or other materials.
2. Bring a member from a local support group to discuss his/her diagnosis.
3. For 'other information' section:
   a. Mention famous people who have had this illness. Use 'People with Mental Illness' poster available from Wellness Reproductions and Publishing, LLC.
   b. Offer list of recommended resources: books, videos, audiotapes
   c. Discuss prevalence, etiology, prognosis
4. Give this handout to a client for him/her to complete after s/he watches a recommended video or listens to an audiotape.
5. Eliminate common myths about mental illness. Use 'Myths and Facts' on page 26 for an additional activity if time allows.

About My Symptoms

A symptom is an indication of an illness. Symptoms can be physical, emotional, perceptual, or seen as a disturbance in thinking. Symptoms can vary from individual to individual even within the same diagnosis. They are signs that an illness may be coming on.

The typical symptoms I experience of my diagnosis, _____,

are _____

_____

_____ .

The earliest symptom I remember having is: _____

_____

_____

_____

Recently, someone noticed that I was having the following symptom:

_____

_____

_____

The most disturbing or irritating symptom is: _____

_____

I will watch for these symptoms as a sign that my illness needs attention:

_____

_____

_____

_____

_____

About My Symptoms

IDEAS FOR HOW-TO-USE

1. Offer concept of symptoms of the flu or a cold prior to the illness, as an example.

2. Emphasize that recognizing early symptoms is an excellent way to prevent an illness from becoming full-blown.

3. Discuss how close family or friends may be able to recognize symptoms, sometimes even before the client does. This feedback can be viewed as supportive if it is said with respect and caring.

4. Present a local volunteer speaker who is in recovery from a mental illness. Ask him/her to discuss how being aware of symptoms may be useful in the recovery process.

About My Medication

My diagnosis is: _____
_____

I take medication: _____
How many times per day?   1   2   3   4   When? _____
What dosage? _____

This medication controls the symptom(s) of: _____
_____
_____

Possible side effects of this medication are: _____
_____
_____

Benefits of this medication are: _____
_____
_____

I *take / do not take* this medication as prescribed. (circle)

I need help in remembering to take my medications correctly.   __Yes __No

If I have questions about my medications, I will _____

Other: _____
_____
_____

About My Medication

IDEAS FOR HOW-TO-USE

1. Distribute one *"About My Medication"* handout for each of the clients' medication.
2. Bring a medication/drug book for reference.
3. Discuss value of pharmacist as part of the health care team.
4. Discuss and compare services of local pharmacies.
5. Review when to call the doctor, and when not to, in regards to running out of meds, side effects, etc.
6. Review prescription information sheet from pharmacy or the Internet.
7. Address concerns about medications and possible addictions.
8. Discuss effects of combining alcohol and prescription medications.
9. Discuss possible risks of discontinuing medications without the assistance of a physician.

About My Coping Strategies

Coping strategies are the tools used to manage an illness. They vary from person to person and can change throughout one's life. Coping strategies might be creative, physical, social, musical, spiritual, intellectual, or fit into another category! They often take time to develop, but are worth the effort as they can make a significant contribution to symptom management.

A coping strategy I used when I was younger: _____
_____
_____

It still works for me _____ doesn't work for me _____.

A coping strategy that I have used lately, that works well for me is:
_____

I learned this skill from: _____

I do this skill _____ times per week.

When I use this strategy, I notice that _____
_____

A coping strategy I am learning that might work is: _____
_____

To manage my symptoms well, I need to do this strategy _____ times per week.

How I can motivate myself to remember to use this strategy is: _____
_____

I hope this strategy will help me by: _____

Using coping strategies can help me by: _____
_____

About My Coping Strategies

IDEAS FOR HOW-TO-USE

1. Generate a list on dry-erase board of all coping strategies observed or taught to this individual / group.

2. Use directly after a successful activity / experience that could be used as a coping strategy.

3 Interview a client about one effective coping strategy.

4. Relate how coping strategies are like tools, and the importance of having enough tools in the 'carpenter's bag' to get the job done.

5. Discuss obstacles to coping strategy development.

6. Discuss coping strategies that participants are aware of, but are not using. Process how these strategies could be helpful.

About My Supports

Supports are vital in managing any illness. Professional supports and personal supports are there to help you when you need it. They can be leaned on when things are challenging or tough. Supports can be reassuring, kind and offer valuable feedback.

Professional supports may include members of the health care team, legal system, spiritual community, etc.

Members of my Professional Support Team include: (name and profession)

_____
_____
_____

They are beneficial to me because: _____

_____
_____

Personal supports may include friends, family, neighbors, members of an organization in which you belong, etc.

Members of my Personal Support Team include: (name and relationship)

_____
_____
_____

They are beneficial to me because: _____

_____
_____

How do you use these supports? _____

_____
_____

About My Supports

IDEAS FOR HOW-TO-USE

1. Emphasize that taking responsibility for one's illness includes developing effective supports.
2. Develop list of situations where supports could be needed. Determine whether individuals have supports needed to handle those situations.
3. Demonstrate in a physical way what supports do.
4. Discuss meaning of "No (wo)man is an island."
5. Discuss obstacles that individuals face in developing and keeping supports.
6. Introduce concept that supportive feedback may include hearing something we don't want to hear, but may be useful in the recovery process.
7. Brainstorm possible additional supports.

About My Supports

About My Strengths

Strength gives us energy to go on.
It helps us come back from setbacks and disappointments.

Strengths are what we do well and what we have going for us.

My physical strengths are: _____

These are important to me because: _____

I do well in: _____

This is important to me because: _____

I do well in: _____

This is important to me because: _____

I have _____ going for me.

This is important to me because: _____

I have _____ going for me.

This is important to me because: _____

Other: _____
_____
_____
_____
_____
_____
_____

About My Strengths

IDEAS FOR HOW-TO-USE

1. Generate list of variety of possible strengths including safe housing, financial, having supports and coping strategies, trusting my doctor, access to medications, legs that walk, insight, good manners, etc.

2. Use as homework sheet allowing others to contribute such as family, friends and staff.

3. Use after a self-esteem or gratitude group.

About My
Area(s) That Need Improvement

It is important to recognize that managing an illness can be complicated. There may be areas interfering with the recovery process. Taking note of personal reflections, monitoring stress levels carefully and considering health care professionals' recommendations may reveal areas that need improvement.

An area that I think needs improvement is: _____

_____

_____ (name of person / people) that would agree.

I realize it's important to improve in this area because: _____

_____

If I don't improve in this area, the consequences might be: _____

_____

Things that get in the way of improving in this area are: _____

_____

Supports, strengths or resources that will help me improve in this area are:

_____

_____

If I improve in this area, I might expect: _____

_____

Other: _____

_____

_____

_____

About My Area(s) That Need Improvement

IDEAS FOR HOW-TO-USE

1. Relate how substance abuse, lack of assertiveness skills, lack of independent living skills, living in a toxic environment, spending time with the 'wrong people.' may be obstacles in recovery.

2. Discuss the topic of insight and its value in recovery.

3. Recognize those who had areas in the past that needed improvement and were able to do so.

About My Resources

There are many resources available to help in the recovery process.

Books: _____
_____
_____

Audiotapes/Videotapes: _____
_____
_____

People: _____
_____
_____

Community Services/Local Organizations: _____
_____
_____

Hotline: _____
_____
_____

National Organization(s): _____
_____
_____

Websites: _____
_____

Other: _____
_____

About My Resources

IDEAS FOR HOW-TO-USE

1. Use in ongoing manner throughout program for clients to collect this information in various ways.
2. Explore websites and free downloads as a way to provide resources.
3. Show favorite books, videos, pamphlets, etc.
4. Bring in speaker from community to describe services offered.

These are the Topics in the Life Management Skills Book Series

Life Management Skills I, II, III, IV, V, VI, VII Topics	LMS I	LMS II	LMS III	LMS IV	LMS V	LMS VI	LMS VII	Total Handouts
• Abuse					3			3
• Activities of Daily Living		2		2			3	7
• Aging			2		2			4
• Anger Management		6						6
• Anxiety/Fear						3	3	6
• Assertion	4	3						7
• Body Image			2					2
• Combating Stigma				2				2
• Communication		4	3	2			3	12
• Conflict Resolution			2					2
• Coping Skills		4	4		8		3	19
• Coping w/ Serious Mental Illness				3				3
• Creative Expression			2			5		7
• Discharge Planning	2							2
• Emotion Identification	2						3	5
• Exercise	3							3
• Feedback			2					2
• Goal Setting	4					2	2	8
• Grief/Loss		3			3			6
• Healthy Living			3		4			7
• Home Management				4				4
• Humor		2		2				4
• Independent Living Skills						3		3
• Interpersonal Skills					2	3		5
• Job Readiness			2	2				4
• Journalizing				3				3
• Leisure	2			4	4	2	2	14
• Life Balance		3						3
• Making Changes					4			4
• Medication Management					4			4
• Money Management		3					2	5
• Motivation	2							2
• Nurturance			4					4
• Nutrition	3							3
• Parenting		2		3	2			7
• Personal Responsibility						2		2
• Positive Attitude					2	3		5
• Problem Solving	3							3
• Productive/Work Activities						2		2
• Recovery/Relapse Prevention		3	2		4	8	5	22
• Relationships		5	4	4	3		2	18
• Reminiscence		3						3
• Responsibility				3			3	6
• Risk Taking	3							3
• Role Satisfaction	2		4					6
• Safety Issues		2						2
• Self-Awareness	3		4					7
• Self-Empowerment			2					2
• Self-Esteem	4	3	2	2	4	2	5	22
• Self-Expression					2			2
• Sexual Health				2				2
• Skill Development							2	2
• Sleep	2							2
• Social Skills			2	2			3	7
• Spirituality						3	3	6
• Stress Management	3	2	3	6		5		19
• Suicide Issues				2				2
• Supports	2	2			2			6
• Therapeutic Treatment						2		2
• Time Management	3	3					4	10
• Values Clarification	3			2				5
TOTAL ACTIVITY HANDOUTS	50	50	50	50	50	50	50	350

7 SELF-MANAGER CARD GAMES Corresponding to 7 LIFE MANAGEMENT SKILLS Books

Use these card games to facilitate development of a variety of Life Management Skills! Since there are more cards than required for a typical 50-minute group session, you can choose the specific topics and cards that would be most beneficial for your intended population and setting.

You can liven up groups with relevant topic cards. Teach by 'DOING'! Use these open-ended cards, integrating knowledge while playing a card game! **Each deck of cards corresponds with one of the Life Management Skills books and has 63 cards & 9 blanks to fill in your own.** In the lower right corner of each card is the page number of its corresponding book. Can be used alone or with corresponding books.

---

18 FOCUS TOPICS including: Discharge Planning, Emotion Identification, Goal Setting, Motivation, Nutrition, Problem Solving, Risk-Taking, Role Satisfaction and more.

Here are some examples from 4 of the other topics:

VALUES CLARIFICATION: *What qualities do you value in the people you deal with regularly (honesty, loyalty, trust, sincerity, intelligence, etc.)?*

STRESS MANAGEMENT: *How do you presently cope with a difficult situation in your life? How can you improve your coping skills?*

SELF-AWARENESS: *When was the last time you truly felt good about yourself? What were the circumstances?*

ASSERTION: *Describe one way you can better communicate with someone important in your life.*

| PRDW-71011 Self-Manager I cards | $15.95 |

---

18 FOCUS TOPICS including: Communication, Grief and Loss, Life-Balance, Money Management, Parenting, Reminiscence, Steps to Recovery and more.

Here are some examples from 4 of the other topics:

TIME MANAGEMENT: *Can you be counted on to be on time? Why or why not?*

SUPPORT SYSTEMS: *Is it easy for you to accept help? Will you ask for help when you need it?*

ANGER MANAGEMENT: *What is something that sparks your anger? How do you handle it?*

SELF-ESTEEM: *When you are given a compliment, do you usually acknowledge or accept it? Do you suggest that you really don't deserve it?*

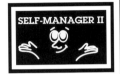

| PRDW-71012 Self-Manager II cards | $15.95 |

---

18 FOCUS TOPICS including: Aging, Body Image, Conflict Resolution, Creative Expression, Feedback, Healthy Living, Nurturance, Self-Empowerment and more.

Here are some examples from 4 of the other topics:

COPING SKILLS: *Have you ever used "writing"... writing letters, journal writing, or poetry - as a way to learn more about yourself or to cope with stress? If yes, describe. If no, would you try?*

RELATIONSHIPS: *Do you feel fatigued after spending time with a certain friend or relative? Who and why?*

JOB READINESS: *What are 3 benefits of women working outside of the home?*

SOCIAL SKILLS: *What is a label, stereotype, or prejudice that offends you? Why?*

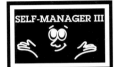

| PRDW-71013 Self-Manager III cards | $15.95 |

---

18 FOCUS TOPICS including: Activities of Daily Living, Serious Mental Illness, Relationships, Responsibility, Sexual Health, Suicide Prevention/Awareness, Values and more.

Here are some examples from 4 of the other topics:

COMMUNICATION: *Name 3 topics that you can talk about with someone you've just met. What are 3 things not to talk about with someone you hardly know?*

JOURNALIZING: *I have learned _____ about my mood/illness/health.*

HUMOR: *Name 3 things, or people, that always make you laugh.*

STRESS MANAGEMENT: *How long do you tend to hold on to anger or hurt feelings? How do you let go?*

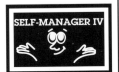

| PRDW-71014 Self-Manager IV cards | $15.95 |

---

15 FOCUS TOPICS including: Coping Skills, Grief, Interpersonal Skills, Leisure, Parenting, Positive Attitude, Self-Expression and more.

Here are some examples from 4 of the other topics:

MEDICATION MANAGEMENT: *What are "over-the-counter" medications for? Compare them with prescription medications.*

MAKING CHANGES: *What are 3 unhealthy eating habits you have?*

RECOVERY: *What are symptoms of your illness that warn you when it may reoccur?*

ABUSE: *If someone asks you to go out with them and your intuition tells you not to, what can you do and say?*

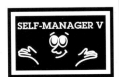

| PRDW-71015 Self-Manager V cards | $15.95 |

---

15 FOCUS TOPICS including: Goal Setting, Healthy Living, Personal Responsibility, Positive Outlook, Relationships, Self-Esteem, Spirituality and more.

Here are some examples from 4 of the other topics:

ANXIETY/FEAR: *Finish the sentence: I am fearful of _____. Explain.*

EXPRESSIVE THERAPY: *If you were a 'super-hero' – what would two of your 'super-skills' be?*

INDEPENDENT LIVING SKILLS: *What benefits are, or would, be important to you in a job?*

THERAPEUTIC TREATMENT: *What role does 'trust' play in your Doctor/Patient relationships? How about your personal relationships?*

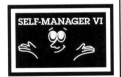

| PRDW-71016 Self-Manager VI cards | $15.95 |

---

18 FOCUS TOPICS including: Productive / Work Activities, Personal Recovery Packet, Skill Development, Social Skills, Money Management, Relapse Prevention and more.

Here are some examples from 4 of the other topics:

ANXIETY: *Who do you feel that you could be more expressive and appreciative towards?*

RECOVERY: *The most frequent excuse I give people when I don't want to do something is _____.*

RESPONSIBILITY: *What is the biggest obstacle you face in taking medications as prescribed?*

COMMUNICATION: *Cross your arms in front of you. Ask group members to interpret what this body language might mean.*

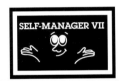

| PRDW-71017 Self-Manager VII cards | $15.95 |

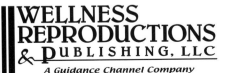

WELLNESS REPRODUCTIONS & PUBLISHING, LLC

A Guidance Channel Company

Call for catalogue 800 / 669-9208 or Fax 800 / 501-8120
email: info@wellness-resources.com
website: www.wellness-resources.com

LMS VII Order Form

SHIP TO:

First Name | Last Name | MI

Title or Initials | Department

Organization/Facility

Street Address | Suite or Apt. No.

City | State | Zip + four

Phone | Fax

E-mail Address

BILL TO:

First Name | Last Name | MI

Title or Initials | Department

Organization/Facility

Street Address | Suite or Apt. No.

City | State | Zip + four

Phone | Fax

E-mail Address

GUARANTEE: Wellness Reproductions & Publishing, LLC stands behind its products 100%. We will refund, exchange or credit your account for the price of any materials returned within 30 days of receipt (excluding shipping). **ALL MERCHANDISE NEEDS TO BE IN PERFECT, RESALE-ABLE CONDITION.** Simply call us at 1-800-669-9208 for a return authorization number.

Order Code	Quantity	Name of Product / Description	Page No.	Price Each	Total Price
PRDW-71007		Life Management Skills VII	–	$ 41.95	
PRDW-71017		Self-Manager VII cards (corresponds with Life Management Skills VII)	–	$ 15.95	
PRDW-71009		Life Management Skills VII book & cards – KIT (value - $57.90)	–	$ 51.95	
PRDW-71008		Life Management Skills I through VII books - KIT (value - $289.65)	–	$ 254.95	
PRDW-71018		Self-Manager I through VII Cards – KIT (value - $111.65)	–	$ 99.95	
PRDW-71019		Life Management Skills I through VII Books & Cards – KIT (value - $401.30)	–	$ 349.95	
PRDW-71898		Medication Management Strategies – 8½" x 11" Handout Pad (50 sheets per pad)	32	$ 9.95	
PRDW-71893		Medication Management Strategies – 24" x 36" Laminated Poster	32	$ 15.95	
PRDW-71896		Medication Management Strategies – 4¼" x 5½" Notepad (50 sheets per pad)	32	$ 3.95	
PRDW-71897		Breaking Down Barriers – 8½" x 11" Handout Pad (50 sheets per pad)	11	$ 9.95	
PRDW-71894		Breaking Down Barriers - 24" x 36" Laminated Poster	11	$ 15.95	
PRDW-71895		Breaking Down Barriers – 4¼" x 5½" Notepad (50 sheets per pad)	11	$ 3.95	

Method of Payment:

☐ Check or money order in U.S. funds.

☐ Purchase Order (must be attached) P.O. #_____

☐ Visa   ☐ MasterCard   ☐ American Express

Print Name _____

Signature _____

Subtotal	
* Shipping and Handling	
Subtotal	
NY and OH Sales Tax	
Grand Total	

Account Number | Expiration Date

See below for Shipping/Handling information.

Easy Ways to Order:

To expedite all orders include order code above.

① **CALL**
Toll-Free:
1/800/669-9208

② **MAIL to:**

Wellness Reproductions & Publishing, LLC
135 Dupont St.
P.O. Box 760
Plainview, NY 11803-0760

③ **FAX**
Toll-Free:
24 hours a day, 7 days a week
1/800/501-8120

④ **ORDER ONLINE:**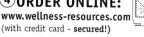
www.wellness-resources.com
(with credit card - **secured!**)

SHIPPING / HANDLING

*REGULAR GROUND:

Add 8% (min. $5.95) in 48 contiguous states.

For Alaska, Hawaii, Puerto Rico, Canada and all other international locations; and for rush, express or overnight delivery, please call for rates and delivery information.

Shipments outside of the United States may be subject to additional handling charges and fees. Customers are responsible for any applicable taxes and duties.

Our Order Policies ensure fast, efficient service!

SALES TAX: New York and Ohio residents, add sales ta on total, including shipping and handling. Tax-exempt organizations, please provide exempt or resale number when ordering.

SHIPPING: We ship all in-stock items withing the contiguous 48 states via UPS or USPS. Back orders are items that are currently out of stock, but will be shipped to you as soon as possible. There is no additional cost for shipping and handling of back orders if shipped separately from your original order. Please allow up to 7-10 working days for delivery.

PRICING: This order form supersedes al previous order forms. Prices subject to change without notice. If this form has expired, we will bill you any difference in price.

UNIVERSITY INSTRUCTOR? If you are considering using this book as a school text or supplemental resource, please call our office to discuss desk copies and quantity education discounts.

METHODS OF PAYMENT:

CHECK: Make your check payable to Wellness Reproductions & Publishing, LLC.

OPEN ACCOUNT: We accept purchase orders from recognized public or private institutions. New accounts please call for information on how to set up an account.

CREDIT CARDS: Please include account number, expiration date and your signature.

UPDATE OUR MAILING LIST: You are automatically added to our mailing list when you order your first product from us. If you want to change your address, remove your name, or eliminate duplicate names from our file, please contact us. We sometimes make available our mailing list to outside parties. If you do not wish to have your information shared, please let us know.

TERMS: Purchase orders, net 30 days.

F.O.B. NY. All international orders must be prepaid in U.S. Funds.

FEEDBACK - LIFE MANAGEMENT SKILLS VII

1. Check the topics that were of special interest to you in LMS VII.

   _____ Activities of Daily Living   _____ Leisure   _____ Responsibility
   _____ Anxiety   _____ Money Management   _____ Self-Esteem
   _____ Communication   _____ Productive/Work Activities   _____ Skill Development
   _____ Coping Skills   _____ Recovery   _____ Social Skills
   _____ Emotions   _____ Relapse Prevention   _____ Spirituality
   _____ Goals   _____ Relationships   _____ Time Management

2. What topics would be of interest in future publications?

   a) _____
   b) _____
   c) _____

3. Which were your favorite handouts?

   a) _____
   b) _____
   c) _____

4. Describe an activity that you have created for any of the pages in this book.

   _____
   _____
   _____

5. Comments on LMS VII: _____

   _____
   _____

If the activity or comments can be published in our WELLNESS NET•WORK newsletter or website, please sign with your professional initials for publication. If it is selected, you will receive a $25 WELLNESS gift certificate.

(signature) _____   (date) _____

Name _____   Title _____
Facility _____   Occupation _____
Address _____   Home Address _____
City _____   City _____
State _____ Zip _____   State _____ Zip _____
Phone (work) (____) _____   Phone (home) (____) _____
email _____   Fax _____

(SEE REVERSE SIDE FOR ORDER FORM)